Relationships and Mental Health

Zoë Boden-Stuart • Michael Larkin
Editors

Relationships and Mental Health

Relational Experience in Distress and Recovery

palgrave
macmillan

Editors
Zoë Boden-Stuart
Faculty of Arts and Social Sciences
The Open University
Milton Keynes, UK

Michael Larkin
College of Health and Life Sciences
Aston University
Birmingham, UK

ISBN 978-3-031-50046-6 ISBN 978-3-031-50047-3 (eBook)
https://doi.org/10.1007/978-3-031-50047-3

Cover illustration: A. Martin UW Photography/ getty images

This Palgrave Macmillan imprint is published by the registered company Springer Nature Switzerland AG.
The registered company address is: Gewerbestrasse 11, 6330 Cham, Switzerland

Paper in this product is recyclable.

Acknowledgements

The editors would like to acknowledge the support of the Independent Social Research Foundation, who funded a research network on 'Relationships and Relatedness in Mental Health' where the initial ideas for this book took shape. We would also like to thank our collaborators in that network: Lisa Bortolotti, Mike Clark, Donna Haskayne, Hanna Pickard, Rex Haigh, Jacqui Gabb and Jerry Tew for their insights. Zoë Boden-Stuart would like to acknowledge the support of the *Care, Health and Emotional Wellbeing* research group at the University of Brighton. Michael Larkin would like to acknowledge the support of the *Phenomenology of Health and Relationships* research group at Aston University.

Contents

Contributors

Humma Andleeb is a lived experience researcher interested in the mental health of minoritised groups and is currently working on her mixed-methods UCL-Wellcome PhD in Mental Health Science.

Nick Benefield is the retired Director of the UK Department of Health National Personality Disorder Programme and was Joint Head of the NHS/ Ministry of Justice Offender Personality Disorder Programme.

Mark Bernard is the lead psychologist for the Birmingham Early Intervention in Psychosis Service, UK. His interests include psychological approaches following first episode psychosis and development of pathways for at-risk mental states.

Zoë Boden-Stuart is Lecturer in Critical and Psychosocial Mental Health at the Open University, UK and is a UKCP-accredited individual and group psychotherapist.

Steven D. Brown is Professor at Nottingham Business School, Nottingham Trent University. His research interests are around social remembering among 'vulnerable' groups, and service user experiences of mental health care.

Divine Charura is Professor of Counselling Psychology and Programme Director for the doctorate in Counselling Psychology at York St John University (England).

Richard Currie is a scholar activist based in Manchester interested in social justice issues relating to disability/mental health with a particular focus on everyday lived experience.

Brian Devlin is a shift coordinator and co-founder of the Worthing Food Foundation, a non-referral community foodbank in West Sussex.

Andy Fox is Assistant Professor at the University of Birmingham and Clinical Psychologist at Birmingham and Solihull Mental Health NHS Foundation Trust. He specialises in recovery from complex and enduring difficulties with psychosis.

Maria Haarmans (PhD) is a trainee clinical psychologist at the University of Liverpool, an Honorary Research Fellow and member of the Centre on the Dynamics of Ethnicity at the University of Manchester.

Gillian Haddock is Professor of Clinical Psychology at the University of Manchester, UK, is the Mental Health theme lead in the Manchester Biomedical Research Centre and an NIHR Senior Investigator.

Fozia Haider has worked across public and voluntary sectors, most recently in public health addressing health inequalities within marginalised communities. She is a passionate Community Bridgebuilder and strives to empower those facing multiple disadvantages.

Rex Haigh is a retired NHS psychiatrist in medical psychotherapy. He is Honorary Professor of Therapeutic Environments at Nottingham University and is involved with several voluntary sector mental health organisations.

Nicola Harrison is a PhD candidate in Psychology and Sociology at The University of Auckland, New Zealand. Her whakapapa is Ngāi Te Rangi and Ngāti Raukawa ki te Waikato on her Father's side and vaka Puaikura from Rarotonga and Urquhart Scottish on her mother's side. A survivor herself, Nicola's work in family sociology explores family relationships through trauma, betrayal and secrecy.

Raj Hazzard respectful rebel dedicated to pulling the margins into focus. Mental health, having been a foe and friend, brings with it the realisation that beyond value judgements lies Shangri-la.

Orly Klein is Senior Lecturer in Psychology at the University of Brighton. Orly's research interests focus on community mental health interventions for people in financial need and service users considered 'hard to reach'.

Michael Larkin is Reader in Psychology at Aston University, in Birmingham. He is a qualitative and phenomenological researcher, with a particular interest in youth and family mental health.

Jade Le Grice is Senior Lecturer in Psychology and Associate Dean Māori in Science at The University of Auckland, New Zealand. Her whakapapa is Ngāpuhi and Te Rarawa on her mother's side and Pākehā (New Zealand European) on her father's side. Also a survivor, Jade's research explores sexual and reproductive health and justice.

Tanya Mackay is Senior Research Manager at McPin. Her work focuses on developing peer research as a methodological approach and ensuring lived experience involvement in all aspects of research.

Charlotte Marriott is Principal Clinical Psychologist working in Early Intervention in Psychosis and At-Risk Mental State services in the Midlands, UK. She has special interests in trauma, EMDR and psychosis.

Andreja Mesarič is an anthropologist and lived experience researcher with an interest in gender and migration. She currently works as a Programme Quality Advisor for the NGO *People in Need*.

Jennie Parker works from a lived experience perspective across research, training and consultation. Recent roles include Lived Experience Development Lead at Berkshire Healthcare NHS and Researcher at City, University of London.

Vanessa Pinfold is co-founder and Research Director at the McPin Foundation (www.mcpin.org) and has worked in mental health research for 30 years both in universities and the voluntary sector.

Dani Plowman is a public health consultant at West Sussex County Council with an interest in food insecurity and wellbeing.

James P. Ravenhill is Lecturer in Psychology at Royal Holloway, University of London. His current research is focussed on intersections of sexuality, masculinity, and health and wellbeing.

Paula Reavey is Professor at London South Bank University, and research and education director of the Design in Mental Health Network. Paula's research and teaching focuses on lived experiences of distress.

Laura Richmond is a researcher and writer with lived experience of autism and complex PTSD. She has a PhD in history and works freelance in a variety of different roles.

Hilary Schan is women's liaison coordinator at the Worthing Food Foundation, a non-referral community foodbank in West Sussex.

Penn Smith is Associate Professor and leads the BA in Counselling and Mental Health and Post-graduate Diploma in Humanistic Counselling at York St John University (England). For Penn's publications see https://urldefense.com/v3/__https://ray.yorksj.ac.uk/profile/2131__;!!NLFGqXoFfo8MMQ!vTMavicteMcvJ7PW8a0yk8NQISlwLaLPGi-vELOzdm7tdzpj2JjKy0Ryxr0IsICyvn9KcraQg2gk9curAyIM8sYP$

Amy Symonds trained as a clinical psychologist at the University of Birmingham. Upon qualifying she worked with adults with long-term physical health problems, and currently works with children, young people and families in Paediatric services in Worcestershire.

Rose Thompson is Senior Research Manager at McPin. She has an interest in narrative and creative research methods and supporting peer researchers in this work.

Kristi Urry is Lecturer in (Critical) Health Psychology and Qualitative Research Methods at the University of Adelaide. Her research interests span sexuality and sexual health, LGBTQIA+ health and person-centred healthcare.

Filippo Varese is Clinical Senior Lecturer in Psychology at the University of Manchester (UK), an NIHR Advanced Research Fellow and the Director of the Complex Trauma and Resilience Research Unit at Greater Manchester Mental Health NHS Foundation Trust.

Carl Walker is a community psychologist from the University of Brighton. As part of the Covid-19 response, he co-founded a local mutual aid group and foodbank charity, The Worthing Food Foundation.

Claire Warrington is a Research Fellow in mental health and policing at the University of York. Both her professional and academic backgrounds have focussed on the lived experience of individuals from marginalised groups and centred around the criminal justice system.

Rebecca White completed her PhD: 'Exploring romantic relationships in the context of psychosis: a mixed methods approach' in 2021. She is now Lecturer in Psychology at the University of Manchester.

Charlotte Wilcox is Lecturer in Counselling Psychology at University of Brighton, UK and is in private practice in the city as an integrative relational UKCP-accredited psychotherapist.

Mary Wise is a volunteer coordinator at the Worthing Food Foundation, a non-referral community foodbank in West Sussex.

List of Figures

List of Tables

Part I

Relationality and Relatedness in the Context of Distress and Recovery: Key Foundations

1

Introduction: Why Relationships Matter for Mental Health

Zoë Boden-Stuart and Michael Larkin

Social approaches to mental health have a long history: social psychiatry and community psychology have, for very many years, argued that the relational context of mental health should be acknowledged. Recently though it has begun to receive wider academic and clinical recognition. The idea for this book began almost ten years ago, with a grant from the Independent Social Research Foundation for a research network on the theme of 'Relationships and Relatedness in Mental Health'. We invited a group of academics from different disciplines to take part in a series of workshops, followed by an event attended by people with lived experience of mental health challenges, practitioners, and academics from psychiatry, psychology, sociology, social work, and beyond. From these conversations, it became clear that whilst there is an abundance of theory

Z. Boden-Stuart (✉)
The Open University, Milton Keynes, UK
e-mail: zoe.boden-stuart@open.ac.uk

M. Larkin
Aston University, Birmingham, UK

Z. Boden-Stuart, M. Larkin (eds.), *Relationships and Mental Health*,
https://doi.org/10.1007/978-3-031-50047-3_1

and robust evidence about the relational context of mental health (as we will explore in the first three chapters of this book), there are still gaps in our knowledge. There is also the challenge of trying to find the relevant literatures siloed within disparate disciplines, each with their own terminology and concepts, and make appropriate links between theory, evidence, policy, and practice. It is into this context, that we offer this edited collection, in the hope that it will draw together some of these threads and provide an interdisciplinary perspective on relational thinking in contemporary adult mental health.

It is well documented that supportive, close relationships are central to wellbeing (e.g. Baumeister & Leary, 1995; Hawkley & Cacioppo, 2010), but connectedness in the context of mental health and distress is complex. Interpersonal relationships are dually implicated in both "the creation and amelioration of mental health problems" (Pilgrim et al., 2009, p. 235). People experiencing distress can sometimes find relationships 'risky' or frightening (Dorahy et al., 2013; Lysaker et al., 2005; Redmond et al., 2010), often in the context of early experiences of trauma and adversity (Edwards et al., 2003; Read et al., 2005), and stigmatisation and exclusion are commonplace (De Silva et al., 2005; Pilgrim et al., 2009; Sayce, 2001). Nevertheless, connectedness is such a fundamental need for most people that, even in challenging circumstances, people desire, seek, or attempt to preserve relational bonds. Where relationships occur and are maintained, they often have a protective effect and support wellbeing. Evidence suggests that romantic relationships (Braithwaite & Holt-Lunstad, 2017) and friendships in adulthood (Pezirkianidis et al., 2023) are particularly important for this. There is also a growing interest in the therapeutic utility of peer-support relationships (where people with lived experience support each other) in mental health contexts (see Shalaby & Agyapong, 2020).

What is less well established is how the person in crisis or distress thinks, feels, and experiences their relational world. Until relatively recently, asking people who had complex mental health needs about their personal experience of relationships was fairly unusual in the context of research, and not much more common within clinical contexts. The lived experience of relationships in the context of mental health is a central focus of this book.

How, when and where relationships take place in the context of psychological distress, and what those relationships feel like for the people involved, can be shaped, at least partially, by how psy-professionals think about relationships and relationality. This includes their ethical views and professional praxis, as well as their personal feelings and thoughts about what relationships should look like and their role in mental health crises. Those professionals work within services, institutions and socio-political contexts that, on the whole, view the person as individual and independent.

Professionals working in mental health are trained in many different ways, but services are typically structured to be psychiatry-led. Psychiatric doctors and nurses are trained in medical models of mental health, which construe distress and other aspects of madness primarily as the result of biological processes, in discrete organisms, albeit with varying degrees of acknowledgement paid to the contribution of psychological and social factors. The issue from a relational point of view is less about the sufficiency of a biomedical model, and more about the limitations of the individualistic assumptions which tend to underpin it. Individualism means that professionals, and the services they work within, struggle to take account of the relational context of distress and recovery. They are further constrained by limited resources, a risk-averse culture, and 'production line' organisational structures (Tew et al., 2015). Often they have no recourse to a reliable repertoire of strategies for incorporating the everyday landscape of relationships into clinical practice. While such strategies require formal co-development and evaluation, one of our hopes for this book is that it might pave the way for such work.

In research, there has been an emerging acknowledgement that connectedness has a fundamental role in recovery (e.g. Marino, 2015; Mezzina et al., 2006; Price-Robertson et al., 2017; Schön et al., 2009; Tew et al., 2012; Topor et al., 2006). In clinical settings too there have been calls to recognise the relational context of distress (e.g. Priebe et al., 2013; Johnson, 2017). Innovative, relationally-focused interventions are emerging and gaining some traction within statutory services in the UK (e.g. Open Dialogue; Seikkula et al., 2006) and elsewhere. At policy level too, there have been indications that relationality and relationships are being taken more seriously (e.g. UK Cabinet Office *Think Family*, 2008;

the UK Care Act, 2014; House of Common's *Tackling Loneliness* briefing, 2019).

However, the "independence imperative" (Taylor, 2015, p. 248) seen in contemporary adult mental health services still predominates, and this means that research and praxis around relationality and distress has been scattered across academic disciplines and siloed within particular groups of practitioners and policy makers. Accounts of the relational complexities facing people who experience distress, their loved ones, and the professionals who work with them, deserve amplification and analysis.It is our aim with this book to start to bring together some of the disparate literature and research that explores these themes. This book draws on a range of disciplinary perspectives, including experiential, community, clinical, and critical psychology; psychotherapy; and social psychiatry. With it, we are attempting to illuminate some of the 'messiness' of relational life in the context of mental health, with the person experiencing distress always at the centre of our endeavours.

This first part of the book, 'Relationality and relatedness in the context of distress and recovery: Key foundations', includes two further chapters that set the scene for the rest of the volume. In *Conceptual foundations: Relational thinking for mental health contexts,* we (Zoë Boden-Stuart and Michael Larkin) give an overview of the theoretical concepts that will act as touchstones throughout the chapters of the book. In its partner chapter, *Clinical foundations: A brief history of relational practice,* Zoë Boden-Stuart and Charlotte Wilcox provide an overview of how relational thinking has permeated, and been excluded from, clinical practice in adult mental health.

The second part of the book 'Relational trauma; relational recovery' comprises three chapters presenting empirical research focused on psychological crisis and complexity, and exploring how relational approaches can help to heal this distress. Nicola Harrison and Jade Le Grice describe how Māori survivors of familial childhood sexual abuse in Aotearoa (New Zealand) draw strength from Māori practices relating to care and reciprocity, spirituality, and collectivity, which support individual healing and bring about change within the family group. Claire Warrington draws on research conducted in England, with women who experience recurrent suicidal distress and are frequently subjected to 'Section 136' detentions by the police. Her work looks at how factors such as relational consistency, trust and understanding can underpin positive experiences with services and break the cycle of suicidal distress. The final chapter in this part by Penn Smith and Divine Charura describes empirical research undertaken with people using a mental health rehabilitation facility and a refugee and asylum seeker service in England. Both groups had experienced significant relational trauma, and the authors argue that it is only by encountering therapeutic and reparative relationships that steps towards recovery can be made. They offer some recommendations for practitioners to guide this work.

The third part of the book 'Peers, family and community: Care and companionship through distress and recovery' offers insights into how relationships with specific others are impacted by, and impact on, mental health needs and experiences. Humma Andleeb and colleagues at the McPin Foundation in the UK, outline the relational values that underpin peer-support in the context of mental health. Charlotte Marriott and colleagues, and Amy Symonds and colleagues offer complementary accounts of relational experience in the context of psychosis. Marriott focuses her chapter on research undertaken with families where one person was under the care of an Early Intervention in Psychosis service. She explores family resilience and strategies for connection and care. Symonds describes research with young people that asks them to consider their relationships through drawing their important connections, and reflecting on how they change over the time of their recovery. The final chapter in this part, from Carl Walker and colleagues, considers mental health outside of clinical settings, in the community context of the current 'cost-of-living crisis' in the UK. The chapter draws on research to show how food insecurity is accompanied by psychological distress, and how food banks can provide an opportunity for relational intervention that supports dignity, solidarity, and connection.

Part IV, 'Love and sex: Negotiating intimacies in mental health settings' includes three chapters that tackle the complexity of how services engage with intimacy. Kristi Urry, writing about the Australian mental health service context, considers how mental health institutions themselves are implicated in a sexuality-related silence, making recommendations for developing training, cultures and research. Rebecca White and colleagues focus on British psychosis services, explorings the ways in which professionals' fears about 'risk' can inhibit opportunities for people to experience romantic relationships in this context. The final chapter in this part, by James Ravenhill and colleagues, looks at another setting where 'risk' becomes paramount. Their chapter explores sex and sexuality in secure forensic mental health wards, where the concept of 'relational security' often overlooks patients' relational desires and experiences with one another.

The final part of the book looks forward. 'New directions: Building a relational approach to distress and recovery' includes Rex Haigh and Nick Benefield's manifesto for a relational practice movement, arguing that change is needed across all staff and services. Our final chapter takes stock of where we are, and where we might hope to be with regard to the integration of relational thinking within clinical and community mental health praxis. We conclude by looking at what is still left to understand when taking a relational perspective to distress and recovery.

References

Baumeister, R. F., & Leary, M. R. (1995). The need to belong: Desire for interpersonal attachments as a fundamental human motivation. *Psychological Bulletin, 117*(3), 497.

Braithwaite, S., & Holt-Lunstad, J. (2017). Romantic relationships and mental health. *Current Opinion in Psychology, 13*, 120–125.

De Silva, M. J., McKenzie, K., Harpham, T., & Huttly, S. R. (2005). Social capital and mental illness: A systematic review. *Journal of Epidemiology & Community Health, 59*(8), 619–627.

Dorahy, M. J., Corry, M., Shannon, M., Webb, K., McDermott, B., Ryan, M., & Dyer, K. F. (2013). Complex trauma and intimate relationships: The impact of shame, guilt and dissociation. *Journal of Affective Disorders, 147*(1–3), 72–79.

Edwards, V. J., Holden, G. W., Felitti, V. J., & Anda, R. F. (2003). Relationship between multiple forms of childhood maltreatment and adult mental health in community respondents: Results from the adverse childhood experiences study. *American Journal of Psychiatry, 160*(8), 1453–1460.

Hawkley, L. C., & Cacioppo, J. T. (2010). Loneliness matters: A theoretical and empirical review of consequences and mechanisms. *Annals of Behavioral Medicine, 40*(2), 218–227.
House of Commons. (2019). *Briefing paper 8514: Tackling loneliness*. House of Commons Library. Available at: https://researchbriefings.parliament.uk/ResearchBriefing/Summary/CBP-8514#fullreport. Accessed 27 Jan 2020.
Johnson, S. (2017). Social interventions in mental health: a call to action. *Social Psychiatry and Psychiatric Epidemiology, 52*(3), 245–247.
Lysaker, P. H., Johannesen, J. K., & Lysaker, J. T. (2005). Schizophrenia and the experience of intersubjectivity as threat. *Phenomenology and the Cognitive Sciences, 4*(3), 335–352. https://doi.org/10.1007/s11097-005-4067-1
Marino, C. K. (2015). To belong, contribute, and hope: First stage development of a measure of social recovery. *Journal of Mental Health, 24*(2), 68–72.
Mezzina, R., Davidson, L., Borg, M., Marin, I., Topor, A., & Sells, D. (2006). The social nature of recovery: Discussion and implications for practice. *Archives of Andrology, 9*(1), 63–80.
Pezirkianidis, C., Galanaki, E., Raftopoulou, G., Moraitou, D., & Stalikas, A. (2023). Adult friendship and wellbeing: A systematic review with practical implications. *Frontiers in Psychology, 14*.
Pilgrim, D., Rogers, A., & Bentall, R. (2009). The centrality of personal relationships in the creation and amelioration of mental health problems: The current interdisciplinary case. *Health, 13*(2), 235–254. https://doi.org/10.1177/1363459308099686
Price-Robertson, R., Obradovic, A., & Morgan, B. (2017). Relational recovery: Beyond individualism in the recovery approach. *Advances in Mental Health, 15*(2), 108–120.
Priebe S, Burns T, Craig TKJ. The future of academic psychiatry may be social. *British Journal of Psychiatry, 2013;202*(5), 319–320. https://doi.org/10.1192/bjp.bp.112.116905
Read, J., van Os, J., Morrison, A. P., & Ross, C. A. (2005). Childhood trauma, psychosis and schizophrenia: A literature review with theoretical and clinical implications. *Acta Psychiatrica Scandinavica, 112*(5), 330–350.
Redmond, C., Larkin, M., & Harrop, C. (2010). The personal meaning of romantic relationships for young people with psychosis. *Clinical Child Psychology and Psychiatry, 15*(2), 151–170. https://doi.org/10.1177/1359104509341447
Sayce, L. (2001). Social inclusion and mental health. *Psychiatric Bulletin, 25*(4), 121–123.

Schön, U. K., Denhov, A., & Topor, A. (2009). Social relationships as a decisive factor in recovering from severe mental illness. *International Journal of Social Psychiatry, 55*(4), 336–347.

Seikkula, J., Aaltonen, J., Alakare, B., Haarakangas, K., Keränen, J., & Lehtinen, K. (2006). Five-year experience of first-episode nonaffective psychosis in open-dialogue approach: Treatment principles, follow-up outcomes, and two case studies. *Psychotherapy research, 16*(02), 214–228.

Shalaby, R. A. H., & Agyapong, V. I. (2020). Peer support in mental health: Literature review. *JMIR Mental Health, 7*(6), e15572.

Taylor, B. (2015). *The last asylum: A memoir of madness in our times.* Hamish Hamilton.

Tew, J., Ramon, S., Slade, M., Bird, V., Melton, J., & Le Boutillier, C. (2012). Social factors and recovery from mental health difficulties: A review of the evidence. *The British Journal of Social Work, 42*(3), 443–460.

Tew, J., Morris, K., White, S., Featherstone, B., & Fenton, S. J. (2015). What has happened to 'Think Family' – Challenges and achievements in implementing family inclusive practice. *Pavilion Annual Parental Mental Health and Child Welfare Work, 1*, 59–64.

Topor, A., Borg, M., Mezzina, R., Sells, D., Marin, I., & Davidson, L. (2006). Others: The role of family, friends, and professionals in the recovery process. *Archives of Andrology, 9*(1), 17–37.

UK Cabinet Office Social Exclusion Task Force. (2008). *Think Family: Improving the life chances of families at risk.* Available at: https://data.parliament.uk/DepositedPapers/Files/DEP2008-0058/DEP2008-0058.pdf. Accessed 31 May 2023.

UK Government. (2014). *Care Act.* Available from: https://www.legislation.gov.uk/ukpga/2014/23/contents/enacted. Accessed 31 May 2023.

2

Conceptual Foundations: Relational Thinking for Mental Health Contexts

Zoë Boden-Stuart and Michael Larkin

This chapter aims to sensitise the reader to relevant relational concepts and ideas that we are loosely referring to as 'relational thinking'. Relational thinking is an assemblage of ideas drawn from extensive literatures across the fields of philosophy, psychology, psychotherapy, sociology and social work, which explore what it means to be inter-connected with others, interpersonally, socially and existentially. In this chapter, we will look at what these concepts and ideas mean more broadly, placing them in the mental health context as a lens for understanding distress and recovery. This chapter, and its partner chapter '*Clinical foundations: A brief history of relational practice*' then provide a jumping-off point for reading the rest of this book.

Z. Boden-Stuart (✉)
The Open University, Milton Keynes, UK
e-mail: zoe.boden-stuart@open.ac.uk

M. Larkin
Aston University, Birmingham, UK

Z. Boden-Stuart, M. Larkin (eds.), *Relationships and Mental Health*,
https://doi.org/10.1007/978-3-031-50047-3_2

Being-With as a Fundamental Aspect of Personhood

In the phenomenological and existential traditions, the *value* and *meaning* of being with others can sometimes be appraised differently, but there is general agreement that there is something *foundational* about the 'withness' of experience. For many phenomenologists, the condition of 'being-with' others (or *mitsein*) is one dimension of the inescapably world-entangled quality of human beings. We cannot escape it; even in solitude, we are still being-with in an existential sense. This relational dimension of being-in-the-world has often been foregrounded by psychologically-minded readings of Heidegger and Merleau Ponty (e.g. see Larkin et al., 2006), and was perhaps first emphasised by the psychiatrist Binswanger, who argued that persons are "fundamentally immersed in a world of human relating" (Frie, 2010, p. 79). This means that—in the Heideggerian sense—one feature of our being is that we are 'thrown' into a world of social relations, structures, language and meanings. The world and person are mutually constitutive, and thus these relational and social aspects of it serve both to afford and shape what we can do, and how we can be. It also means that—after Gadamer—one condition of being is that we continually have to strive to be understood *by* (and in turn, *to u*nderstand) other persons. We can think of this as a dialogical condition—after Buber—by emphasising that, while mutuality is a primary feature of human experience, it is achieved through an effortful process, mediated by culture, language and social structures (Carel, 2013). Binswanger goes further than his phenomenological sources, and argues that through the condition of being-with, an authentic connection with others can be the basis for therapeutic change (Frie, 2010). He is concerned with the work that has to be done to achieve such change, and he begins by emphasising the importance of understanding the other's world, as they experience it. This is a first step for the therapist. It is also a stance shared in many of the contributions to this book, which set out to describe (and then reflect upon) what a relational experience of mental distress is *like*, from the point of view of the people who are striving to understand it. It is no coincidence that empathy was one of the earliest topics chosen for detailed phenomenological study (Stein, 1917), because an understanding of empathy is central to progressing our understanding of each other, and of our relationality (Meneses & Larkin, 2012).

It is also common to see that attending to the intersubjective nature of human existence often leads to a further focus on care and ethics, as we see for example in the literature on lifeworld-led healthcare (Todres et al., 2007). This is also evident in some of the work in this volume, which takes the logical next step, and asks 'if our shared experiences are like *this,* then what would an appropriately caring and helpful response look like?'

These early phenomenological writers, and their subsequent psychological and psychiatric 'translators', have set out some key conceptual foundations for understanding relationality as a central component of the human condition, and of humans' ability to cope with that condition. A range of contributions and developments have built upon these foundations, so that we also have more fine-grained conceptual tools for understanding some of the ways in which our relational experiences are: shaped by early life experiences; given meaning via emotion; and implicated in our moral responsibilities towards others. To take these one at a time, early life experiences are implicated in setting some of our individual 'parameters' for intersubjective engagement (see below, on attachment). This is important, because to live well, we need to be able to find acceptable forms of *attunement* between ourselves and the other people who are important to us. Such attunements are relational, reciprocal and dynamic (i.e. it is not simply that some people are 'better' at attunement than others), but our ability to achieve meaningful connections with others is—in part—shaped by what we have already learned about how to understand ourselves, and how to understand others (Fonagy et al., 2015). The emphasis on learning is important here: people continue to learn throughout the life course, and new modes of relating and connecting can be supported by a range of personal and professional relationships. This links tidily to the second point: emotional experiences are an important tool for signalling and receiving meaning with regard to relationships, and we can develop our abilities to understand this. Researchers in the field of enactive and embodied cognition have written of the world as 'affectively scaffolded' for us (Krueger, 2020) and of people as 'affectively entangled' with one another (e.g. see Casey, 2022). These ideas develop directly from Edith Stein's early phenomenological analysis of empathy as a direct and non-intellectual insight into the experience of another (Colombetti, 2014). Contemporary readings of the empathy concept, and of the ways in which humans connect with one another more generally, are made more complex by insights into neurodiversity, and specifically by research on autism and the 'double empathy' problem (Milton et al., 2023). This perspective highlights the challenges of 'cross-neurotype' communication, and questions the framing of autism as a type of 'social deficit', pointing towards the many important ways in which autistic people do seek and value experiences of mutuality. This means that we need to be mindful of differences in the way that relationality develops and manifests, and to be ready to support and nurture connectedness in its many forms.

One conceptual framing in contemporary phenomenological writing seems particularly helpful for supporting this kind of complexity. Edward Casey has argued that emotions are not the exclusive, interior property of the subject—but rather are embodied, enacted and available in the space between people—and thus that we can think of the empathising subject as someone who is actively feeling *into* the experience of another (Casey, 2022). It is not inconsistent with this position to suggest that different expectations of another's orientation towards the world might arise from our own orientation towards the world.

What we might also notice here is that our relational lives place us in a position of vulnerability or precariousness with regard to both other individuals (Butler, 2009) and organisations (Carel & Kidd, 2021). Others may reciprocate in ways which we find sustaining and supportive, or they may react in ways which we find threatening and harmful. Such vulnerability requires an ethical discussion about our responsibility towards each other, and the care that we owe each other.

Philosophical writing on the implications of a second-person perspective (Darwall, 2009) has drawn out the nature of our moral obligations as being fundamentally interpersonal in nature. The concept of care ("the fact that people look after one another, take care of one another and thus are responsible"; Laugier, 2016, p. 207) is pivotal. Laugier argues that because care is 'ordinary', and taken-for-granted, it tends to be overlooked and devalued—and she draws on the work of the developmental psychologist Carol Gilligan to exemplify and develop this point (Laugier, 2018; Gilligan, 1982). Gilligan is a key figure in the foregrounding of the relational focus in psychology. Her work on moral development identifies the individualist conceptual and methodological assumptions embedded within psychological theories of development. She shows how these tend to overvalue abstract individualist principles as indicators of successful maturation, and to overlook the nuance of the more grounded, relational praxis which actually allows society to function. Both Gilligan and Laugier are working from a feminist standpoint, and thus an important element of their critique is that what gets made 'visible' is highlighted because it is implicated in the reproduction of patriarchal norms. These ideas are important because they describe some of the structural challenges we face when we attempt to prioritise relations of care over individual responsibilities and needs.

Understanding Relational Experience from a Developmental Perspective

A number of psychological concepts describe how various aspects of people's relational capabilities are shaped in early life, and develop into adulthood. These concepts—intersubjectivity, attachment, belonging, trust—are also connected to some experiences of distress, and to some of the ways in which people may experience the actions of families, professionals and services in response to that distress.

Across the life course, relationships contribute to the development and maintenance of a sense of self and identity, and to people's capacity to cope with (and reflect upon) difficult experiences. Psychological research has shown that the building blocks for our capacity to relate to others are laid very early in life. Drawing on phenomenological ideas and empirical studies with infants, child psychologist Colwyn Trevarthan (1998) developed a theory of innate intersubjectivity which argues that the infant has 'other-awareness'. Building on observational studies which show that reciprocal emotional exchange forms part of the earliest interactions with caregivers, the innate intersubjectivity theory argues that we are born with intrinsic motivations towards companionship and cooperation. These motives extend beyond survival needs, and suggest that understanding the infant's "purposeful intersubjectivity or an initial psychosocial state" is fundamental for understanding how mental health and wellbeing develop in the growing person (Trevarthen & Aitken, 2001, p. 3). We can track this back to the phenomenological work about how relatedness and intersubjectivity are fundamental features of personhood, and also link it forward, to connect with higher-level concepts such as belonging (see below).

Attachment is one important mechanism which helps us to understand how people experience and achieve their relatedness to others, and how we might begin to explain some of the individual differences which characterise people's varying modes of relating to one another. Attachment theory suggests that different attachment styles (expectations and beliefs about the self, and what it is due from others) are established in infancy—as per Bowlby's and Ainsworth's classic experimental studies—according to how the child experiences their primary caregiver's emotions, especially in situations where there is uncertainty and threat (Main, 2000). These styles, and their development into adulthood, have complex implications for how people experience and manage their adult relationships. For example, some attachment styles are associated with poor emotional regulation (Girme et al., 2021; Mikulincer & Shaver, 2019; Mortazavizadeh & Forstmeier, 2018), which in turn mediate between attachment and some adult mental health diagnoses (Lewczuk et al., 2021; Peng et al., 2021). Similarly, attachment may shape how we interact with professionals and services (Blackburn et al., 2010). In turn, this means that thinking about attachment is important for the design and delivery of mental health services (Bucci et al., 2015), and for the conduct and experience of mental health workers themselves (Linington, 2020).

Building on this, Baumeister and Leary (1995) trace their own argument from Bowlby, but also from Freud, Maslow and others in the Western psychotherapeutic canon. They argue that humans have a fundamental need to belong. More specifically, they suggest that: we need frequent non-aversive emotional interactions within at least one stable and reciprocal interpersonal relationship; that we are motivated strongly by this need; that we will readily seek out, create, and maintain such relationships whenever possible; and that failure to find or keep these relationships has considerable physical and mental health repercussions. More recently they have revised their theory to include the need to be accepted and belong within groups, as well as with individuals (Allen et al., 2022). Developmentally, this is a process that is typically navigated during adolescence and early adulthood, as people begin to locate and identify themselves in relation to interests and relationships beyond the family. It is this sense of belonging—feeling integral to, and personally involved in, a social system—that Hagerty and colleagues (1992) referred to when they noted how often mental health nurses heard patients saying they didn't fit in, weren't important to anyone or didn't feel part of anything. Reviews have shown how a sense of belonging is central to a good quality of life for people experiencing mental health needs (Connell et al., 2012), and that it is one of a number of mechanisms that link social connectedness to improvements in health and wellbeing (Thoits, 2011).

Trust is implicated in each of these framings. Trust is both a dynamic mechanism for judging the safety of relationships (e.g. it may be afforded by others, or it may not) and a resource which can be depleted, and replenished. Trust is important throughout the life course because of its role in situating and evaluating our relationships with others. People receiving psychiatric diagnoses are far more likely than others to have been exposed to adverse childhood experiences, which often include betrayals of trust, such as abuse, violence and neglect (e.g. Bebbington et al., 2011; Read & Bentall, 2012). This can mean that in later life, people find it more difficult to trust others, or make poor judgements regarding who or how much to trust, leaving them more vulnerable to abusive behaviour from others. As with attachment, issues of trust are likely to be important for service design and delivery (Brown et al., 2009; Gaebel et al., 2014). In particular, the negative impact of poor practices may be especially amplified for people for whom trust is already difficult.

Theorists have argued that our motivation for connectedness is innate and highly influential in shaping our behaviour. Psychological and psychotherapeutic research with infants and adults has shown that the specific conditions of our early relational life shape our understandings and expectations of others, including how safe and trusting we may feel with significant others in our lives, and with mental health professionals.

The Contrasting Experiences and Consequences of Intimacy and Loneliness

As we have shown, intersubjectivity is unavoidable: we seek social connection for our physical and psychic survival. However, *how* we interact—to what extent we feel close to or distanced from others—depends on a range of contextual factors, characteristics, desires and opportunities. These modulations in intimacies and solitudes are so fundamentally implicated in our wellbeing, that some have suggested that mental health diagnoses amount to a "pathology of intersubjectivity" (Di Petta et al., 2022, p. 203).

Intimacy refers to closeness and connection between people, which can be bodily (e.g. sexual experience, affection), emotional (e.g. love), behavioural (via the 'practices of intimacy'; Morgan, 2009) and/or cognitive (e.g. shared values, or being 'of like mind') (Jamieson; 2011). Intimacy typically involves people feeling special to one another, and sharing significant levels of trust, attachment, familiarity and privileged knowledge (Jamieson, 2005). From this definition, intimacy sounds optimistic, but in intimacy there are also:

> the unavoidable troubles, distractions and disruptions [...] Romance and friendship inevitably meet the instabilities of sexuality, money, expectation, and exhaustion, producing, at the extreme, moral dramas of estrangement and betrayal, along with terrible spectacles of neglect and violence even where desire, perhaps endures. (Berlant, 1998, p. 281)

Intimacy therefore is messy, painful and unpredictable, and yet, it is something that we all generally strive for. It is also not solely a private matter, but also a public one. Through the discourses and regimes of 'therapisation', psychologisation, and medicalisation, intimacies are shaped by our health and legal systems (Berlant, 1998). We do our best to demarcate our intimate relationships from other social encounters through 'boundary work', but intimacy has a habit of leaking into domains that we do not typically think of as places of intimacy. Where and when intimacies intersect with mental health settings is particularly fraught. Mental health services are not well set-up to acknowledge that, for most human beings, sexuality and emotional closeness are fundamental to living. Intimacy is closely related to mental health recovery (Boucher et al., 2016) and is also a human right (Hicks, 2016), yet people with mental health diagnoses have intimacy needs that are typically unmet (McCann, 2010). This is most likely because intimacy in mental health services is usually associated with 'risk', which becomes a barrier to providing support, especially when mixed with prejudicial ideas about the relational needs of people with certain diagnoses (White et al., 2019).

Intimacy can also include caregiving and being cared for, or about. Informal care, the sort that happens within families and across broader social networks, is complex (Barnes, 2012), but increasingly in the mental health context, this is where the majority of care is happening. The relational contexts in which care occurs has been overlooked (Moyneaux et al., 2011) and instead, researchers have focused considerable effort on understanding the 'burden' of caring for someone with mental health needs (see Cham et al., 2022). This literature considers both the objective (e.g. picking up medications) and subjective (e.g. feeling worried) 'burdens' of the caring relationship, which can be considerable: caring for someone with complex mental health needs can result in family members becoming psychologically distressed themselves (e.g. Savage & Bailey, 2004; Mittendorfer-Rutz et al., 2018). Family relationships where there are mental health issues often become strained (Corcoran et al., 2007), and they are more likely to involve difficult or ambivalent feelings compared to the general population (Randolph, 1998). This type of interpersonal conflict and emotional distance within family relationships is a significant source of distress for the person with mental health needs (Griffiths et al., 2019).

Reciprocity in caring relationships has tended to be somewhat overlooked, and caregiving and care-receiving have often been viewed as mutually exclusive (Guest & Corrigan, 2018). However, some studies have looked at how people with complex mental health needs contribute and care for others within their networks (e.g. Allman et al., 2018; Boden-Stuart et al., 2021; Coldwell et al., 2011). Reciprocity is also, of course, a key feature of peer support relationships and recovery programmes (e.g. Tanaka & Davidson, 2015).

Non-familial relationships in the context of mental health are under-researched. Taking psychosis as an example, we do know that people's social networks tend to include twice as many family members as friends (Palumbo et al., 2015), and that relationships with friends and romantic partners suffer during crises (e.g. Macdonald et al., 2005), and can be perceived as 'risky' by the person in distress (Redmond et al., 2010). In the case of psychosis, deficits in social cognition (Bertrand et al., 2007) or specific mental health experiences like paranoia (Freeman et al., 2002), or social anxiety (Michail & Birchwood, 2010) have been put forward as reasons why friendships and romantic relationships may fail. Fear and prejudice can also cause people to distance themselves from the person in crisis, although evidence suggests that social distancing is reducing, perhaps due to policy attempts to address mental health stigma in the UK (Robinson & Henderson, 2019). Hospitalisation can also disrupt relationships, where wards act as a physical and psychological barrier to closeness (Fenton et al., 2014; Hickman et al., 2016; Horan et al., 2006). Stable friendships are known to protect against the impact of stressors, but conflictual, unequal or antagonistic friendships increase distress (King et al., 2016). However, because of the positive 'buffering' effect of increased social support, services sometimes try to engineer social relationships. One way this happens is via befriending programmes, but these can be confusing for service-users: a 'befriender' is a professionalised and boundaried role that appears to be very different from what a person in distress expects from a friend (Thompson et al., 2016).

Whilst intimacies are painful and complex, especially so in the context of mental health, their opposites are perhaps even more painful. A number of concepts could be grouped together under the theme of social disadvantage, which is both a cause and consequence of poor mental health (Morgan et al., 2007). Loneliness, social isolation, social exclusion, social rejection, social distance, social capital, marginalisation, stigmatisation and discrimination are all relevant concepts when thinking about how poor relational experiences at interpersonal and structural levels impact on mental health outcomes. Unsurprisingly, there have been several calls for more conceptual clarity in the literature (e.g. Morgan et al., 2007; Wang et al., 2017), with terms coming in and out of vogue with policymakers. Most recently in the UK, loneliness appears to have captured policy imaginations (e.g. House of Commons, 2019; Department for Digital, Culture, Media & Sport, 2018).

Loneliness has been described as the psychological equivalent of hunger; a "social pain", with probable evolutionary origins aiming to motivate the maintenance of social connectedness for the benefit of the collective (Cacioppo et al., 2006, p. 1056). Loneliness refers to the subjective perception or feeling of isolation, rather than the objective state of being isolated, and feeling lonely is extremely common across the population (Hawkley & Cacioppo, 2010). It can come about from distortions in our attunement or co-regulation with others, such that our desires and actions to reach out are missed, or misunderstood, or our judgements on the balance of sharing are off-kilter (Galanaki, 2023). In this way, loneliness brings us out of rhythm with others and disrupts our capacity to make shared meaning (Galanaki, 2023). Hawkley and Cacioppo (2010) argue that the feeling of loneliness acts in the same way as feeling physically unsafe, setting off a chain of implicit hypervigilance, activating cognitive biases and raising the expectation that others are a source of threat. Reciprocal behavioural responses in others may then fulfil the expectation of social distance, resulting in a self-perpetuating "loneliness loop" (Hawkley & Cacioppo, 2010, p. 4), wherein neurobiological responses (i.e. stress/threat responses that lead to emotional dysregulation) and behavioural mechanisms (i.e. coping strategies like substance misuse) together contribute to poor physical and mental health outcomes.

Loneliness has been associated with a wide range of poor physical health, cognitive, and mental health outcomes (Hawkley & Cacioppo, 2010) and premature mortality (Holt-Lunstad et al., 2015). There is also a huge literature exploring loneliness and its relevance for mental health (see Heinrich & Gullone, 2006; Wang et al., 2018), and it is well-established that it is implicated in depression and anxiety (Park et al., 2020) and suicide (McClelland et al., 2020). There are now many interventions aiming to tackle the loneliness 'epidemic' (see Mann et al., 2017), though these focus on people who are *already* lonely. An early intervention approach might instead focus on improving very early relationship contexts (e.g. attachment with caregivers) and reducing social disadvantage.

Social Disadvantage and Mental Health

Social isolation (i.e. having fewer social connections) could happen through choice, but perhaps most typically in the case of mental health, it comes about through social disadvantage. Some people more than others are likely to struggle to create or maintain relational connections, and people with mental health issues, particularly psychosis-type experiences, are among the most socially excluded in the UK (Boardman, 2011). A socially excluded person is someone who cannot engage with, or participate in, the activities of their society, because of material, cultural, social or other disadvantage or deprivation (Boardman, 2011; Morgan et al., 2007). People with complex mental health needs are more likely to: be unemployed; be less involved in social groups; live alone; live in more disadvantaged areas; be on benefits; and have immigrant status (Morgan et al., 2007). These conditions all limit or disrupt opportunities for social engagement. Socio-economic disadvantages like these, both during childhood (Reiss, 2013) or adulthood (Thompson et al., 2022) are associated with poorer mental health. Intersectional complexities mean that those with minoritised identities, because of race, class, sexual orientation or gender, and who also experience mental health needs may face 'multiple jeopardy' (Fagrell Trygg et al., 2019). As with loneliness, there are robust associations between social isolation and poorer mental health outcomes (e.g. Leigh-Hunt et al., 2017): smaller social networks are more common for people with complex mental health needs and, in turn, these are associated with more frequent hospitalisations (Albert et al., 1998). Our relational networks, and the trust we place in them, act as a resource on which we can draw at times of need (Morgan et al., 2007). When this 'social capital' (Putnam, 2000; Morgan et al., 2007) is reduced, the outcome is also poorer mental health (Ehsan et al., 2019). Poor mental health also leads to social disadvantage.

Stigma and discrimination diminish social trust and increase isolation. Mental health stigma and discrimination are persistent and pervasive, and their consequences, including shame and isolation, are often experienced as more distressing and disabling than the mental health condition itself (Thornicroft et al., 2022). Stigma operates at interpersonal and structural levels, creating barriers to fulfilment in personal (via self-stigma), relational and occupational domains (Thornicroft et al., 2022, p. 1438). At the structural level, stigma has constrained funding and diminished political, academic and clinical interest in mental health resulting in a significant lack of parity with physical health (Vigo, 2016). In addition, people with mental health diagnoses have much poorer physical health and earlier mortality than those without, due to the 'diagnostic overshadowing' of certain mental health diagnoses, and institutional and personal prejudices. Stigma is also a *cause* of poor mental health. For example, minority stress theory posits that LGBTQ+ people internalise discrimination and prejudice, placing them under unique stressors that explain their poorer mental health compared to heterosexual populations (Meyer, 2003). Psychosocial stressors, like discrimination and their intersections with other forms of adversity and prejudice, cascade across a life course (Nurius et al., 2013), and can cause intergenerational trauma (Fortuna et al., 2022). At an interpersonal level, stigma causes distress, shame and social distancing. An emerging literature identifies mental health-related microaggressions (a term originally related to 'subtle' racist insults and invalidations; see Sue, 2010) as one form of stigmatisation. Both race-related and mental health-related microaggressions are founded on the prejudicial assumption of dangerousness and inferiority, however, the 'perpetrators' of mental health-related microaggressions are most typically family, friends and professionals (Barber et al., 2020).

However, while relationships with others can be made more difficult due to stigma, there are also ways in which understanding and developing a language for talking about one's mental health can be very important from a relational point of view. For example, while worries about stigma and trust may deter help-seeking, *knowledge* about mental health difficulties may facilitate it (e.g. see Radez et al., 2021). In some settings (e.g. amongst young people) stigma may be reduced when there are expectations that mental health difficulties are common and normal (e.g. see Hermann et al., 2022). When help-seeking leads to diagnosis, various studies have shown that—even for the most controversial and disputed and diagnoses, such as Borderline Personality Disorder—people will generally report at least *some* benefits in terms of understanding their experiences and needs, and of being able to explain them to others (e.g. see Horn et al., 2007). These kinds of disclosures to others can be experienced as positive and helpful (e.g. as enhancing the sense of being understood and belonging to a community) when the person making the disclosure has control over the context and purpose of the disclosure (e.g. see Bril-Barniv et al., 2017). These positive benefits may be especially strong for those sharing their experiences in the context of recovery or survivorship communities, via mental health activism, or in the role of lived experience researchers or consultants (e.g. see Gupta et al., 2023). The mental health literacy of *others*—friends, family, employers, health professionals—is also very important for the affordance of positive relational support, and so many psychoeducation interventions target these populations. Interventions which involve family in this way are often amongst the most effective (e.g. see Bighelli et al., 2021; Rodolico et al., 2022) for reducing risk of relapse.

Conclusions

In this chapter we have outlined some of the ways in which being-with others is a fundamental aspect of personhood, and we have described some of the key concepts involved in understanding how our capacity for relational experience develops. We have highlighted the contrasting experiences and consequences of both intimacy and loneliness, and underscored the important role that social inequalities may have for relatedness and mental health. We hope it is clear throughout that there is a co-constitutive relationship between mental health and relatedness: poor mental health often inhibits our opportunities for relational engagement at interpersonal and structural levels; limited opportunities for connection with others, or poor relationships (e.g. high in conflict or low reciprocity), will in turn impact upon our mental health. Thus, relationships and mental health are inextricably intertwined.

Relational thinking offers an important lens for understanding experiences of distress and recovery, and the services and contexts that aim to support mental health and wellbeing, whilst keeping these concepts in mind. The concepts we have outlined here are not exhaustive, and are introduced only briefly—but we hope that readers will find them useful for contextualising and comparing the contributors' chapters in this book, and perhaps to guide their own next steps in working with a relational focus.

References

Albert, M., Becker, T., Mccrone, P., & Thornicroft, G. (1998). Social networks and mental health service utilisation—A literature review. *International Journal of Social Psychiatry, 44*(4), 248–266.

Allen, K. A., Gray, D. L., Baumeister, R. F., & Leary, M. R. (2022). The need to belong: A deep dive into the origins, implications, and future of a foundational construct. *Educational Psychology Review, 34*(2), 1133–1156.

Allman, J., Cooke, A., Whitfield, B., & McCartney, M. (2018). "It doesn't mean I'm useless": How do young people experiencing psychosis contribute to their families and why are contributions sometimes overlooked? *Psychosis, 10*(1), 11–21.

Barber, S., Gronholm, P. C., Ahuja, S., Rüsch, N., & Thornicroft, G. (2020). Microaggressions towards people affected by mental health problems: A scoping review. *Epidemiology and Psychiatric Sciences, 29*, e82, 1–11. https://doi.org/10.1017/S2045796019000763

Barnes, M. (2012). *Care in everyday life: An ethic of care in practice*. Policy Press.

Baumeister, R. F., & Leary, M. R. (1995). The need to belong: Desire for interpersonal attachments as a fundamental human motivation. *Psychological Bulletin, 117*(3), 497.

Bebbington, P., Jonas, S., Kuipers, E., et al. (2011). Childhood sexual abuse and psychosis: Data from a cross-sectional national psychiatric survey in England. *British Journal of Psychiatry, 199*, 29–37.

Berlant, L. (1998). Intimacy: A special issue. *Critical Inquiry, 24*(2), 281–288.

Bertrand, M. C., Sutton, H., Achim, A. M., Malla, A. K., & Lepage, M. (2007). Social cognitive impairments in first episode psychosis. *Schizophrenia Research, 95*(1–3), 124–133. https://doi.org/10.1016/j.schres.2007.05.033

Bighelli, I., Rodolico, A., García-Mieres, H., et al. (2021). Psychosocial and psychological interventions for relapse prevention in schizophrenia: A systematic review and network meta-analysis. *The Lancet Psychiatry, 8*(11), 969–980.

Blackburn, C., Berry, K., & Cohen, K. (2010). Factors correlated with client attachment to mental health services. *The Journal of Nervous and Mental Disease, 198*(8), 572–575.

Boardman, J. (2011). Social exclusion and mental health–how people with mental health problems are disadvantaged: An overview. *Mental Health and Social Inclusion, 15*(3), 112–121.

Boden-Stuart, Z. V., Larkin, M., & Harrop, C. (2021). Young adults' dynamic relationships with their families in early psychosis: Identifying relational strengths and supporting relational agency. *Psychology and Psychotherapy: Theory, Research and Practice, 94*(3), 646–666.

Boucher, M.-E., Groleau, D., & Whitley, R. (2016). Recovery and severe mental illness: The role of romantic relationships, intimacy, and sexuality. *Psychiatric Rehabilitation Journal, 39*(2), 180–182.

Bril-Barniv, S., Moran, G. S., Naaman, A., Roe, D., & Karnieli-Miller, O. (2017). A qualitative study examining experiences and dilemmas in concealment and disclosure of people living with serious mental illness. *Qualitative Health Research, 27*(4), 573–583.

Brown, P., Calnan, M., Scrivener, A., & Szmukler, G. (2009). Trust in mental health services: A neglected concept. *Journal of Mental Health, 18*(5), 449–458.

Bucci, S., Roberts, N. H., Danquah, A. N., & Berry, K. (2015). Using attachment theory to inform the design and delivery of mental health services: A systematic review of the literature. *Psychology and Psychotherapy: Theory Research and Practice, 88*, 1–20. https://doi.org/10.1111/papt.12029

Butler, J. (2009). Performativity, precarity and sexual politics. AIBR. *Revista de Antropología Iberoamericana, 4*(3).

Cacioppo, J. T., Hawkley, L. C., Ernst, J. M., Burleson, M., Berntson, G. G., Nouriani, B., & Spiegel, D. (2006). Loneliness within a nomological net: An evolutionary perspective. *Journal of Research in Personality, 40*(6), 1054–1085.

Carel, H. (2013). *Illness*. Acumen.

Carel, H., & Kidd, I. J. (2021). Institutional opacity, epistemic vulnerability, and institutional testimonial justice. *International Journal of Philosophical Studies, 29*(4), 473–496. https://doi.org/10.1080/09672559.2021.1997393

Casey, E. S. (2022). *Turning emotion inside out: Affective life beyond the subject.* Northwestern University Press.

Cham, C. Q., Ibrahim, N., Siau, C. S., Kalaman, C. R., Ho, M. C., Yahya, A. N., Visvalingam, U., Roslan, S., Rahman, F. N. A., & Lee, K. W. (2022). Caregiver burden among caregivers of patients with mental illness: A systematic review and meta-analysis. *Healthcare, 10*(12), 2423.

Coldwell, J., Meddings, S., & Camic, P. M. (2011). How people with psychosis positively contribute to their family: A grounded theory analysis. *Journal of Family Therapy, 33*(3), 353–371. https://doi.org/10.1111/j.1467-6427.2010.00513.x

Colombetti, G. (2014). *The feeling body: Affective science meets the enactive mind.* MIT press.

Connell, J., Brazier, J., O'Cathain, A., Lloyd-Jones, M., & Paisley, S. (2012). Quality of life of people with mental health problems: A synthesis of qualitative research. *Health and Quality of Life Outcomes, 10*(1), 1–16.

Corcoran, C., Gerson, R., Sills-Shahar, R., Nickou, C., McGlashan, T., Malaspina, D., & Davidson, L. (2007). Trajectory to a first episode of psychosis: A qualitative research study with families. *Early Intervention in Psychiatry, 1*, 308–315. https://doi.org/10.1111/j.1751-7893.2007.00041.x

Darwall, S. (2009). *The second-person standpoint: Morality, respect, and accountability*. Harvard University Press.

Department for Digital, Culture, Media & Sport. (2018). *A connected society: A strategy for tackling loneliness.* Available at: https://www.gov.uk/government/publications/a-connected-society-a-strategy-for-tackling-loneliness. Accessed 31 May 2023.

Di Petta, G., Tittarelli, D., & Vanacore, R. (2022). Mental illness as a pathology of intersubjectivity. In M. Biondi, A. Picardi, M. Pallagrosi, & L. Fonzi (Eds.), *The clinician in the psychiatric diagnostic process* (pp. 203–231). Springer.

Ehsan, A., Klaas, H. S., Bastianen, A., & Spini, D. (2019). Social capital and health: A systematic review of systematic reviews. *SSM-Population Health, 8*, 100425.

Fagrell Trygg, N., Gustafsson, P. E., & Månsdotter, A. (2019). Languishing in the crossroad? A scoping review of intersectional inequalities in mental health. *International Journal for Equity in Health, 18*(1), 1–13.

Fenton, K., Larkin, M., Boden, Z. V., Thompson, J., Hickman, G., & Newton, E. (2014). The experiential impact of hospitalisation in early psychosis: Service-user accounts of inpatient environments. *Health & Place, 30*, 234–241. https://doi.org/10.1016/j.healthplace.2014.09.013

Fonagy, P., Luyten, P., & Allison, E. (2015). Epistemic petrification and the restoration of epistemic trust: A new conceptualization of borderline personality disorder and its psychosocial treatment. *Journal of Personality Disorders, 29*, 575–609.

Fortuna, L. R., Tobón, A. L., Anglero, Y. L., Postlethwaite, A., Porche, M. V., & Rothe, E. M. (2022). Focusing on racial, historical and intergenerational trauma, and resilience: A paradigm to better serving children and families. *Child and Adolescent Psychiatric Clinics, 31*(2), 237–250.

Freeman, D., Garety, P. A., Kuipers, E., Fowler, D., & Bebbington, P. E. (2002). A cognitive model of persecutory delusions. *British Journal of Clinical Psychology, 41*(4), 331–347. https://doi.org/10.1348/014466502760387461

Frie, R. (2010). A hermeneutics of exploration: The interpretive turn from binswanger to gadamer. *Journal of Theoretical and Philosophical Psychology, 30*(2), 79–93.

Gaebel, W., Muijen, M., Baumann, A. E., Bhugra, D., Wasserman, D., Van der Gaag, R. J., Heun, R., & Zielasek, J. (2014). EPA guidance on building trust in mental health services. *European Psychiatry, 29*(2), 83–100.

Galanaki, E. (2023). Loneliness and intersubjectivity: A view from Trevarthen's theory. *Frontiers in Psychology, 14*, 1145739.

Gilligan, C. (1982). *In a different voice: Psychological theory and Women's development.* Harvard University Press.

Girme, Y. U., Jones, R. E., Fleck, C., Simpson, J. A., & Overall, N. C. (2021). Infants' attachment insecurity predicts attachment-relevant emotion regulation strategies in adulthood. *Emotion, 21*(2), 260.

Griffiths, R., Mansell, W., Edge, D., & Tai, S. (2019). Sources of distress in first-episode psychosis: A systematic review and qualitative metasynthesis. *Qualitative Health Research, 29*(1), 107–123. https://doi.org/10.1177/1049732318790544

Guest, C., & Corrigan, O. (2018). Extraordinary normalcy: Home, relationships and identities in narratives of care. *Home and Place, 53*, 71–78. https://doi.org/10.1016/j.healthplace.2018.07.008

Gupta, V., Eames, C., Golding, L., et al. (2023). Understanding the identity of lived experience researchers and providers: A conceptual framework and systematic narrative review. *Research Involvement Engagement, 9*, 26. https://doi.org/10.1186/s40900-023-00439-0

Hagerty, B. M., Lynch-Sauer, J., Patusky, K. L., Bouwsema, M., & Collier, P. (1992). Sense of belonging: A vital mental health concept. *Archives of Psychiatric Nursing, 6*(3), 172–177.

Hawkley, L. C., & Cacioppo, J. T. (2010). Loneliness matters: A theoretical and empirical review of consequences and mechanisms. *Annals of Behavioral Medicine, 40*(2), 218–227.

Heinrich, L. M., & Gullone, E. (2006). The clinical significance of loneliness: A literature review. *Clinical Psychology Review, 26*(6), 695–718.

Hermann, V., Durbeej, N., Karlsson, A.-C., & Sarkadi, A. (2022). Feeling mentally unwell is the "new normal". A qualitative study on adolescents' views of mental health problems and related stigma. *Children and Youth Services Review., 143*, 106660. https://doi.org/10.1016/j.childyouth.2022.106660

Hickman, G., Newton, E., Fenton, K., Thompson, J., Boden, Z. V., & Larkin, M. (2016). The experiential impact of hospitalisation: Parents' accounts of caring for young people with early psychosis. *Clinical Child Psychology and Psychiatry, 21*(1), 145–155. https://doi.org/10.1177/1359104515581716

Hicks, H. (2016). To the right to intimacy and beyond: A constitutional argument for the right to sex in mental health facilities. *NYU Review of Law and Social Change, 40*, 621–673.

Holt-Lunstad, J., Smith, T. B., Baker, M., Harris, T., & Stephenson, D. (2015). Loneliness and social isolation as risk factors for mortality: A meta-analytic review. *Perspectives on Psychological Science, 10*(2), 227–237.

Horan, W. P., Subotnik, K. L., Snyder, K. S., & Nuechterlein, K. H. (2006). Do recent-onset schizophrenia patients experience a "social network crisis"? *Psychiatry: Interpersonal and Biological Processes, 69*(2), 115–129. https://doi.org/10.1521/psyc.2006.69.2.115

Horn, N., Johnstone, L., & Brooke, S. (2007). Some service user perspectives on the diagnosis of borderline personality disorder. *Journal of Mental Health., 16*(2), 255–269.

House of Commons. (2019). *Briefing paper 8514: Tackling loneliness.* House of Commons Library. Available at: https://researchbriefings.parliament.uk/ResearchBriefing/Summary/CBP-8514#fullreport. Accessed 27 Jan 2020.

Jamieson, L. (2005). Boundaries of intimacy. In S. Cunningham-Burley & L. McKie (Eds.), *Families in society: Boundaries and relationships* (pp. 189–206). Policy Press.

Jamieson, L. (2011). Intimacy as a concept: Explaining social change in the context of globalisation or another form of ethnocentricism? *Sociological Research Online, 16*(4), 151–163.

King, A. R., Russell, T. D., & Veith, A. C. (2016). Friendship and mental health functioning. In M. Hojjat & A. Moyer (Eds.), *The psychology of friendship* (pp. 249–266). Oxford University Press.

Krueger, J. (2020). Schizophrenia and the scaffolded self. *Topoi, 39*, 597–609.

Larkin, M., Watts, S., & Clifton, E. (2006). Giving voice and making sense in interpretative phenomenological analysis. *Qualitative Research in Psychology, 3*(2), 102–120.

Laugier, S. (2016). Politics of vulnerability and responsibility for ordinary others. *Critical Horizons, 17*(2), 207–202.

Laugier, S. (2018). Cavell on feminism and the ethics of care. *Conversations: The Journal of Cavellian Studies, 6*, 55–80.

Leigh-Hunt, N., Bagguley, D., Bash, K., Turner, V., Turnbull, S., Valtorta, N., & Caan, W. (2017). An overview of systematic reviews on the public health consequences of social isolation and loneliness. *Public Health, 152*, 157–171.

Lewczuk, K., Kobylińska, D., Marchlewska, M., Krysztofiak, M., Glica, A., & Moiseeva, V. (2021). Adult attachment and health symptoms: The mediating role of emotion regulation difficulties. *Current Psychology, 40*, 1720–1733.

Linington, M. (2020). The significance of the clinician's felt experience. In K. Berry, S. Bucci, & A. N. Danquah (Eds.), *Attachment theory and psychosis: Current perspectives and future directions*. Routledge.

MacDonald, E., Sauer, K., Howie, L., & Albiston, D. (2005). What happens to social relationships in early psychosis? A phenomenological study of young people's experiences. *Journal of Mental Health, 14*(2), 129–143.

Main, M. (2000). Recent studies in attachment: Overview, with selected implications for clinical work. In S. Goldberg, R. Muir, & J. Kerr (Eds.), *Attachment theory: Social, developmental and clinical perspectives*. Routledge.

Mann, F., Bone, J. K., Lloyd-Evans, B., Frerichs, J., Pinfold, V., Ma, R., Wang, J., & Johnson, S. (2017). A life less lonely: The state of the art in interventions to reduce loneliness in people with mental health problems. *Social Psychiatry and Psychiatric Epidemiology, 52*, 627–638.

McCann, E. (2010). Investigating mental health service user views regarding sexual and relationship issues. *Journal of Psychiatric and Mental Health Nursing, 17*, 251–259. https://doi.org/10.1111/j.1365-2850.2009.01509

McClelland, H., Evans, J. J., Nowland, R., Ferguson, E., & O'Connor, R. C. (2020). Loneliness as a predictor of suicidal ideation and behaviour: A systematic review and meta-analysis of prospective studies. *Journal of Affective Disorders, 274*, 880.

Meneses, R., & Larkin, M. (2012). Edith Stein and the psychological study of empathy. *Journal of Phenomenological Psychology, 43*, 151–184.

Meyer, I. H. (2003). Prejudice, social stress, and mental health in lesbian, gay, and bisexual populations: Conceptual issues and research evidence. *Psychological Bulletin, 129*(5), 674.

Michail, M., & Birchwood, M. (2010). Social anxiety in psychosis: Towards a new understanding of affective dysfunction. *Mind and Brain, the Journal of Psychiatry, 1*(1).

Mikulincer, M., & Shaver, P. R. (2019). Attachment orientations and emotion regulation. *Current Opinion in Psychology, 25*, 6–10.

Milton, D., Waldock, K. E., & Keates, N. (2023). Autism and 'the double empathy problem'. In F. Mezzenzana & D. Peluso (Eds.), *Conversations on empathy: Interdisciplinary perspectives on imagination and radical othering* (1st ed.). Routledge.

Mittendorfer-Rutz, E., Rahman, S., Tanskanen, A., Majak, M., Mehtälä, J., Hoti, F., Jedenius, E., Enkusson, D., Leval, A., Sermon, J., Taipale, H., & Tiihonen, J. (2018). Burden for parents of patients with schizophrenia—A nationwide comparative study of parents of offspring with rheumatoid arthritis, multiple sclerosis, epilepsy, and healthy controls. *Schizophrenia Bulletin, 45*, 794–803.

Molyneaux, V., Butchard, S., Simpson, J., & Murray, C. (2011). Reconsidering the term 'carer': A critique of the universal adoption of the term 'carer'. *Ageing Society, 31*(3), 422–437. https://doi.org/10.1017/S0144686X10001066

Morgan, D. (2009). *Acquaintances: The Space Between Intimates And Strangers: The Space Between Intimates and Strangers*. McGraw-Hill Education (UK).

Morgan, C., Burns, T., Fitzpatrick, R., Pinfold, V., & Priebe, S. (2007). Social exclusion and mental health: Conceptual and methodological review. *The British Journal of Psychiatry, 191*(6), 477–483.

Mortazavizadeh, Z., & Forstmeier, S. (2018). The role of emotion regulation in the association of adult attachment and mental health: A systematic review. *Archives of Psychology, 2*(9).

Nurius, P. S., Uehara, E., & Zatzick, D. F. (2013). Intersection of stress, social disadvantage, and life course processes: Reframing trauma and mental health. *American Journal of Psychiatric Rehabilitation, 16*(2), 91–114.

Palumbo, C., Volpe, U., Matanov, A., Priebe, S., & Giacco, D. (2015). Social networks of patients with psychosis: A systematic review. *BMC Research Notes, 8*(1), 1–12. https://doi.org/10.1186/s13104-015-1528-7

Park, C., Majeed, A., Gill, H., Tamura, J., Ho, R. C., Mansur, R. B., ... & McIntyre, R. S. (2020). The effect of loneliness on distinct health outcomes: A comprehensive review and meta-analysis. *Psychiatry Research, 294*, 113514.

Peng, W., Liu, Z., Liu, Q., Chu, J., Zheng, K., Wang, J., Wei, H., Zhong, M., Ling, Y. & Yi, J. (2021). Insecure attachment and maladaptive emotion regulation mediating the relationship between childhood trauma and borderline personality features. *Depression and Anxiety, 38*(1), 28–39.

Putnam, R. D. (2000). *Bowling alone: The collapse and revival of American community*. Simon and Schuster.

Radez, J., Reardon, T., Creswell, C., et al. (2021). Why do children and adolescents (not) seek and access professional help for their mental health problems? A systematic review of quantitative and qualitative studies. *European Child & Adolescent Psychiatry, 30*, 183–211.

Randolph, E. T. (1998). Social networks and schizophrenia. In K. T. Mueser & N. Tarrier (Eds.), *Handbook of social functioning in schizophrenia* (pp. 238–246). Allyn Bacon.

Read, J., & Bentall, R. P. (2012). Negative childhood experiences and mental health: Theoretical, clinical and primary prevention implications. *The British Journal of Psychiatry, 200*, 89–91.

Redmond, C., Larkin, M., & Harrop, C. (2010). The personal meaning of romantic relationships for young people with psychosis. *Clinical Child Psychology and Psychiatry, 15*(2), 151–170. https://doi.org/10.1177/1359104509341447

Reiss, F. (2013). Socioeconomic inequalities and mental health problems in children and adolescents: A systematic review. *Social Science & Medicine, 90*, 24–31.

Robinson, E. J., & Henderson, C. (2019). Public knowledge, attitudes, social distance and reporting contact with people with mental illness 2009–2017. *Psychological Medicine, 49*, 2717–2726. https://doi.org/10.1017/S0033291718003677

Rodolico, A., Bighelli, I., Avanzato, C., et al. (2022). Family interventions for relapse prevention in schizophrenia: A systematic review and network meta-analysis. *The Lancet Psychiatry, 9*(13), 211–221.

Savage, S., & Bailey, S. (2004). The impact of caring on caregivers' mental health: A review of the literature. *Australian Health Review, 27*(1), 111.

Stein, E. (1917/1989). *On the problem of empathy* (W. Stein, Trans.). ICS Books.

Sue, D. W. (2010). *Microaggressions and marginality: Manifestation, dynamics, and impact*. Wiley.

Tanaka, K., & Davidson, L. (2015). Reciprocity in the clubhouse context. *International Journal of Psychosocial Rehabilitation, 19*(2), 21–33.

Thoits, P. A. (2011). Mechanisms linking social ties and support to physical and mental health. *Journal of Health and Social Behavior, 52*(2), 145–161.

Thompson, R., Valenti, E., Siette, J., & Priebe, S. (2016). To befriend or to be a friend: A systematic review of the meaning and practice of "befriending" in mental health care. *Journal of Mental Health, 25*(1), 71–77.

Thompson, R. M., Kopasker, D., Leyland, A., Pearce, A., & Katikireddi, S. V. (2022). Effects of poverty on mental health in the UK working-age population: Causal analyses of the UK household longitudinal study. *International Journal of Epidemiology, 52*(2), 512–522.

Thornicroft, G., Sunkel, C., Aliev, A. A., Baker, S., Brohan, E., El Chammay, R., … & Winkler, P. (2022). The Lancet Commission on ending stigma and discrimination in mental health. *The Lancet, 400*(10361), 1438–1480.

Todres, L., Galvin, K., & Dahlberg, K. (2007). Lifeworld-led healthcare: Revisiting a humanising philosophy that integrates emerging trends. *Medical Health Care Philosophy, 10*, 53–63.

Trevarthen, C. (1998). The concept and foundations of infant intersubjectivity. In S. Braten (Ed.), *Intersubjective communication and emotion in early ontogeny* (pp. 15–46). Cambridge University Press.

Trevarthen, C., & Aitken, K. J. (2001). Infant intersubjectivity: Research, theory, and clinical applications. *The Journal of Child Psychology and Psychiatry and Allied Disciplines, 42*(1), 3–48.

Vigo, D. (2016). The health crisis of mental health stigma. *Lancet, 3*, 171–178.

Wang, J., Lloyd-Evans, B., Giacco, D., Forsyth, R., Nebo, C., Mann, F., & Johnson, S. (2017). Social isolation in mental health: A conceptual and methodological review. *Social Psychiatry and Psychiatric Epidemiology, 52*, 1451–1461.

Wang, J., Mann, F., Lloyd-Evans, B., Ma, R., & Johnson, S. (2018). Associations between loneliness and perceived social support and outcomes of mental health problems: A systematic review. *BMC Psychiatry, 18*(1), 1–16.

White, R., Haddock, G., & Varese, F. (2019). Supporting the intimate relationship needs of service users with psychosis: What are the barriers and facilitators? *Journal of Mental Health, 29*(3), 314–320.

3

Clinical Foundations: A Brief History of Relational Practice

Zoë Boden-Stuart and Charlotte Wilcox

This chapter aims to map how and where relational thinking sits within adult mental health care. It provides a partner chapter to *'Conceptual foundations: Relational thinking for mental health contexts'.* Together these chapters act as a jumping off point for reading the rest of this book. This short chapter is necessarily partial, with its focus on Western psychotherapeutic legacies and, predominantly on the British mental health system, with its very particular way of understanding what it means to be psychologically well. Our chapter starts by giving a brief history of the therapeutic relationship and its links to the importance of early relationships for good mental health. We will then consider the 'independence imperative' within contemporary British (and many Western) adult mental health settings, thinking about how and why praxis and policy that integrates relational thinking seems to be failing to change the

Z. Boden-Stuart (✉)
The Open University, Milton Keynes, UK
e-mail: zoe.boden-stuart@open.ac.uk

C. Wilcox
University of Brighton, Brighton, East Sussex, UK

Z. Boden-Stuart, M. Larkin (eds.), *Relationships and Mental Health*,
https://doi.org/10.1007/978-3-031-50047-3_3

individualistic focus of adult mental health care. We will then explore whether there has been or could be a paradigm shift in contemporary mental health practice within the UK. Finally, we will chart some of the innovations and alternatives that recognise the integral place of relationships and relatedness in mental health experiences, care, and settings.

The Relationship as Therapeutic

Perhaps the most fundamental concern within psychotherapeutic practice is the therapeutic relationship. From Freud onwards, there has been an understanding that distress can be explored, reduced and even resolved through the developing relationship between client and psychotherapist. Research has robustly upheld this view, showing that it is the therapeutic relationship, above all else, that heals (Norcross, 2019; Norcross & Wampold, 2011). This understanding is trans-theoretical, crossing the divide between psychoanalytically and humanistically-informed therapeutic modalities. Classical Freudians envisioned the psychoanalyst as sleuth, embarking on an archaeology of the client's earliest experiences of infancy and family life, using the tools of analysis to reveal the genesis of unconscious conflicts. This investigation uncovered the client's template for relating that would characterise, and when dysfunctional blight, later relationships (Fairburn, 1952; Gomez, 1997). Early humanistic approaches (e.g. following Carl Rogers), however, synthesised American political ideals with the radically democratic counter-cultural ideas emerging in the post-war disillusionment with modernism, and fused Western individualism with Eastern spiritual influences from Buddhist and Hindu mysticism. Humanists saw the therapeutic relationship as a crucible, within which human potential could be realised (Rogers, 1951). The third major development in Western psychotherapeutic practice was cognitive therapy (e.g. following Aaron Beck), where the therapeutic relationship is centred primarily around the task of learning. Cognitive therapy sees a therapeutic relationship (in the style of Rogers) as important but not sufficient for change to take place (Beck, 1976), and views the therapeutic relationship as a space for collaboration, active engagement, and exploratory pedagogical dialogue (Beck, 2020). Despite their differences, all these modalities understood that the potential for change lay in how client and therapist were in relationship with one another.

As psychotherapeutic theory developed, understandings of how the therapeutic relationship worked became more nuanced. In the mid-twentieth century, psychiatrists, and particularly object relations psychoanalysts, progressed our understanding of how early development impacts on later relational life, and with that came new insights into how the therapeutic relationship can heal. Donald Winnicott (1958) argued that emotional wellbeing requires 'good enough' caregiving in early life. 'Good enough' caregiving, is the ordinary to-ing and fro-ing of parenting, in which the caregiver mirrors the child's feelings, and reflects them back, thus helping the child to make sense of themselves. This mirroring creates a special kind of bonding, experienced by the baby as 'holding'. Holding is emotional as much as it is physical, and it creates that felt sense of safety which underpins healthy emotional development. Coupled with the literature on attachment that shows how a caregiver becomes a secure base for a child to explore their world (Bowlby, 2005/1988), this foundational work laid the basis not only for our understanding of what can go well, or not, in early childhood, but also how therapists can utilise these relational qualities within the therapeutic relationship.

The healing quality of the therapeutic relationship is well-established, and the rich history of psychotherapeutic theory and practice has provided numerous insights into the importance of the relationship between caregiver and child, and between therapist and client, many of which are now supported by neuroscientific evidence. However, as we will explore, the uptake of these ideas in mainstream mental health care has not been straightforward.

The "Independence Imperative" in Adult Mental Health Services

The picture that emerges from psychotherapeutic theory points rather uncomplicatedly towards the importance of nurturing 'good enough' relationships between the person and the professionals they work with, as well as between the person and the important others in their lives. It is perhaps surprising then, that mainstream contemporary adult mental health practice, in the UK at least, maintains a dogged focus on independence and individualism (Priebe et al., 2013). In this next section, we will look at how that has come about. There is a great deal of heterogeneity across services in the UK, and it is hard to know exactly what is happening 'on the ground' or how much of what is discussed in research, guidelines, and policies is taken up by services and individual professionals. However, drawing on a few examples from British practice and policy, we will attempt to illuminate some of the barriers that seem to get in the way of services utilising what we know about the positive nature of therapeutic relationships, and relationships more broadly (see *'Conceptual foundations: Relational thinking for mental health contexts'*).

The last asylum in the UK closed in 1993 and UK psychiatric services were shifted into a period of 'community care'. Services, like therapeutic communities and day hospitals, that were based on an understanding that relationships healed, began to close as social psychiatry declined and clinicians began to focus more on the individual (Priebe et al., 2013). In her memoir, 'The Last Asylum', the historian Barbara Taylor describes an *"independence imperative"* (2015, p. 248) in British contemporary adult mental health services. She argues that one legacy of the asylum system is the view that depending on others is indicative of emotional weakness. Mental health professionals and policymakers seem to adhere to this view, and many service-users themselves, she suggests, have also internalised the idea that independence is a marker of 'recovery', and, conversely, that needing others is a sign of illness. Taylor's own experience as a patient in the last asylum in the UK, as well as day centres and outpatient services, informs her arguments, which she also develops from accounts of other survivors of the psychiatric system in the 1970s and 1980s. Deinstitutionalisation and the move to 'community care' that was supposed to support service-users, quickly became replaced with a 'recovery' agenda that prioritised brief, structured one-to-one interventions. Ongoing relationships with staff became much harder to maintain, and with the closure of shared services like day centres, opportunities for interaction with other service-users have also diminished. The independence ideology Taylor describes coincides with years of intense funding cuts for mental health that have decimated services (and continue to do so at this time). A long period of austerity, the exacerbating effects of Covid-19, and more recently the cost-of-living crisis, have reduced statutory and community services to the bare bones (Care Quality Commission, 2022). The development of stepped-care models means that 'self-help', in the form of online psychoeducation and CBT-driven work packages, are now a common first-step treatment option for prescribing clinicians, reducing opportunities for human connection even further.

The health economic focus on individualism extends to how staff interact with one another, and to the relational support available within the mental health system more broadly. Working in mental health settings has always been demanding because of the levels of distress inherent in the work, however, contemporary issues including staff shortages, high workload, and service cutbacks have resulted in a particularly challenging context, where staff burnout and retention are major issues (Long et al., 2023; UNISON, 2017). At the same time, there has been a shift in culture from shared clinical and ethical responsibility to an audit-based culture of managerialism. This disrupts practitioners' attempts to sustain mutual support and to create spaces for reflection and collaboration (Moth, 2020), which impacts on care directly and indirectly. A managerial culture diminishes time for relational engagement with service-users, whilst also failing to support staff to process their emotional responses to their work, reducing their capacity to offer good-enough care. One example of a relational mechanism that can work to help people process and make sense of the anxieties that inevitably arise in mental health care is the reflective practice group. These regular, multi-disciplinary group meetings are spaces where clinical staff are encouraged to share the sometimes-challenging feelings evoked by their work. Relational support like this allows the complex feelings that come up in clinical work to be 'held' (in the Winnicottian sense) and metabolised by the group. This protects the individual from having sole responsibility for trying to make sense of these feelings alone, with the inevitable possibility that the distress is not 'contained' and it spills back into the clinical work. Such group-level intervention supports co-regulation at a nervous-system level, and consequently, attendance at reflective practice groups is associated with lower levels of staff burnout and with higher levels of resilience

(Sadusky & Spinks, 2022). Unfortunately, opportunities for nursing staff to attend consistent, supportive and high-quality reflective practice groups are limited (Topping & Gamble, n.d.) and there are calls for greater investment in staff with the skills to provide reflective practice, clinical supervision, and post-incident debriefing (Ebrahim & Wilkinson, 2021).

A managerial culture has also led to distress becoming synonymous with risk, which then becomes another process to be managed. Hinshelwood and Skogstad (2000) argue that once risk begins to dictate the prevailing managerial logic, effective relational therapeutic work is no longer viable. It is perhaps no surprise then, that psychotherapeutic practice—grounded in the importance of the human relationship—has been consistently withdrawn from mainstream adult mental health practice. Hinshelwood predicted this in 1994 (p. 287) when he argued that psychotherapy was a "potentially subversive activity within the psychiatric service" precisely because it invites, *requires*, emotional responsiveness between people. It is this relational activity—the lively contact between people—that he argued, the psychiatric system was defending against for fear that the 'madness' should overwhelm staff and patients alike. What provision there now is within the NHS for psychotherapy (i.e. for people unable to pay private fees) has been "reduced to a very limited number of sessions of behavioural and other manualized therapy", whilst the more well-off and well-informed can access long-term psychotherapy via private practice, creating a two-tier system (Atkinson, 2023, p. 373). Rizq (2012) has argued that the UK's Improving Access to Psychological Therapies programme (that promised to increase counselling and CBT provision), was overwhelmed by a fetishisation of managerial processes and governance that served to mask the reality that there are limits to the care we are able to provide, and the feelings of helplessness this brings. Rizq and Jackson (2019) argue that the model, with its industrialised approach to care and focus on surveillance and manualisation, dehumanises both clients and therapists. From this policy perspective, the relationship no longer appears to matter.

In spite of all the evidence to suggest that the therapeutic relationship is *the* agent for change, there has been a consistent stripping away of relationally-grounded practices in statutory mental health services. In the

UK, ever-increasingly neoliberal politics and policies, a financial crash, a pandemic, and an inflation crisis have conspired to consolidate the shift towards individualism and independence that Taylor (2015) describes. Both people who use services, and the people who work within them, seem to have succumbed to structures and discourses that erode opportunities for interdependency, emotional vulnerability, and mutuality.

A Paradigm Shift? Towards a Relational Practice

At the same time as relational practice with mental health services has diminished, arguments in support of recognising the role of relational life in mental health have been gathering momentum within academia. In psychiatry and psychology, researchers have long argued that the dominant biomedical approach to understanding mental health was limited, and that attending to the psychosocial underpinnings of distress was imperative for providing effective support. The development of the Adverse Childhood Experiences (ACE) scale (Felitti et al., 1998) led to numerous studies evidencing the causal role of interpersonal ACEs, such as abuse and neglect, in a range of poor mental health outcomes (see e.g. Sheffler et al., 2020). In the 2010s, two influential editorials in the *British Journal of Psychiatry* argued that psychiatry had lost its way, and that the dominant focus on neurobiology had "stifled creativity" in research (Priebe et al., 2013, p. 319) and led to a neglect of the "ethical and hermeneutic aspects" of practice (Bracken et al., 2012, p. 432).

In psychology, a similar shift from an individualising cognitive approach to mental health to a more social and relational approach seems to have taken place. The publication of the British Psychological Society (BPS)'s *The Power, Threat, Meaning Framework* (Johnstone & Boyle, 2018) provided an alternative to psychiatric diagnosis and emphasised the interpersonal, cultural, and social experiences at the heart of understanding and treating distress. Two more recent publications from the BPS, *Understanding Psychosis and Schizophrenia* (Cooke, 2017) and *Understanding Depression* (Bowden et al., 2020) also foregrounded the relational and social underpinnings of distress. An increased recognition of the role of interpersonal and social trauma in complex mental health presentations, and a nuanced understanding of the interplay between trauma, neurobiology, and distress—such as in Read et al.'s (2001, 2014) traumagenic neurodevelopmental theory for psychosis—along with a growing evidence-base for the role of social relationships in supporting (or inhibiting) recovery (Tew et al., 2012), has further supported calls for a paradigm shift towards (or back to) a more relationally-oriented mental health model.

Attempts have been made to bring relational thinking more explicitly into UK policy and practice. UK policy papers and clinical guidelines have, since at least the turn of the millennium, sought to recognise the role of significant others in the care and recovery of a distressed person, and attempted to include them within mental health care. Guidance is scattered across the grey literature, and primarily refers to the 'carer', a contentious term for many in that it implies dependency (Stanbridge & Burbach, 2007), which as Taylor (2015) argues is at odds with the 'independence imperative' of contemporary mental health discourses. Policies to date maintain a narrow focus on a single, family carer, rather than considering the complete network of significant others (family or otherwise) who care for, *and are cared for by*, a person who is distressed (Morris et al., 2008). However, we know that interdependency and reciprocal caring relationships are just as important for those who are struggling with their mental health as for everyone else (see, e.g. Boden-Stuart et al., 2021). Various initiatives and organisations have attempted to bridge the gaps between services, the people who use them, and their loved ones. The Carers Trust/Royal College of Nursing's (Hannan, 2013) best practice guide "The Triangle of Care" looked at how the person in distress, their loved ones, and services could work together. They argued that mental health services needed to be 'carer aware' and to work in partnership with service-user's loved ones. Information sharing is a particularly thorny issue, with family members suggesting that confidentiality is used as a blanket excuse for services not engaging with significant others.

In England, there are clinical guidelines that recommend family interventions, and there are a number of whole-family approaches currently in use within statutory services, including systemic family therapy, family group conferencing, and behavioural group or couple therapy (Tew et al., 2015). In practice, these often only exist only in specialist services (e.g. learning disabilities and substance misuse settings; see Morris et al., 2008 for a review) or within social work contexts (where whole-family work is much more typical), and usually only when there are children in the family. The most common form of family intervention in statutory adult mental health practice seems to be single or multi-family intervention in the form of psychoeducation, perhaps with some behavioural approaches integrated. The UK's clinical guidance for group intervention within adult mental health includes psychosis (family interventions that focus on crisis management, education and support) and depression or bipolar disorder (behavioural couple therapy). Systemic family therapy for adults does have a good evidence base for efficacy across a range of mental health issues (von Sydow et al., 2010; Pinquart et al., 2016), and does remain part of some clinical psychology training programmes. However, in adult mental health care practice, systemic thinking seems to mostly inform service development rather than direct clinical work. Except privately, systemic family therapy is rarely available to adults experiencing mental health-related distress.

Whilst whole-family approaches are struggling to maintain a foothold in adult mental health care, individual therapies that hold relational issues in mind have made some in-roads, although the field is still dominated by CBT. Cognitive Analytic Therapy (CAT; Ryle, Leighton & Pollock, 1997; Ryle & Kerr, 2020), Interpersonal Therapy (IPT; Klerman & Weissman, 1994) and Dynamic Interpersonal Therapy (DIT; Lemma et al., 2011) are examples of brief, structured therapies that retain a specific focus on the clients' relational experiences. CAT is recommended in clinical guidelines for diagnoses of anorexia and borderline personality disorder, however, it is at risk of being 'squeezed out' of NHS provision (Waft, 2011), at least partly because the evidence base is not seen as credible enough for clinical guideline recommendations (Calvert & Keller, 2014). IPT is recommended for depression, and DIT was rolled out as part of IAPT services and has an emerging evidence base for depression (e.g. Fonagy et al., 2020). All these approaches are time limited, reducing the opportunity for the therapeutic relationship to develop. Another area where relational thinking is making somewhat of an impact is within crisis care. Planning who to reach out to in a crisis (significant others and professionals) is a key part of safety planning (Stanley & Brown, 2008), and clinical guidance recommends that significant others should be involved in crisis planning in the case of self-harm and suicide, where the person wants that, and where it is appropriate (NICE, 2022, 2023). In practice, implementing this guidance seems challenging, however, local policies do reflect the wish to include significant others in the development of safety and relapse prevention plans (e.g. Mersey Care, 2019; Oxford Health, 2018) and there is also third sector support for this way of working (Samaritans, n.d.).

Elsewhere in mental health services, relational thinking has been integrated into new models of care. For example, Assertive Outreach Teams (Marshall & Lockwood, 1998; Tyrer, 2000) integrated principles from attachment theory to create a new community psychiatry case management approach. These specialist teams managed complex care needs in the community, aiming to provide a seamless care service for those who were regularly in crisis. Taking an attachment perspective, a designated case worker provided a quasi-therapeutic relationship, and funding was in place for activities that would help to build the relational bond. However, this relationship building was always in tension with the more coercive requirements of role, for example, persuading service-users to take medication where this was dictated by mental health legislation. Reduced bed occupancy rates justified the funding initially, but quickly assertive outreach services were squeezed by financial constraints, whilst disappointing outcome research, and attempts to 'shore up' traditional community services that were under threat, eventually led to their demise (Firn, 2007; Firn et al., 2013).

Despite the clear evidence that relational trauma and social conditions underpin many mental health needs, and despite psychotherapeutic theory and practice increasingly moving towards relational understandings of how therapeutic work happens, adult mental health services in the UK seem to struggle to integrate relational thinking into their care work. Relational thinking keeps re-emerging in policy and practice initiatives, with the impetus coming from the perspectives of the person in crisis, their loved ones, and clinicians themselves. However, relational approaches—whether that is at group, family, or even at the individual level—do not seem to become a core feature of how British mental health services (currently) work.

Relational Alternatives and Innovations

On the peripheries of the mainstream mental health services, through private and charitable organisations, and in some places within the NHS too, alternative, and innovative approaches to relational working are still flourishing.

Therapeutic communities (Main, 1946; Rappoport, 1960; Jones, 1968) have been used to treat complex mental health for at least 50 years (Haigh, 2017). At its simplest, a therapeutic community is a place where "living [t]here is the therapy" (Johnson & Haigh, 2010, p. 30). These group-based treatment modalities involve a flattened hierarchy where staff and patients live alongside one another, with democratisation and shared responsibility, and open enquiry into the meaning and communicatory power of behaviour (Pearce & Haigh, 2017). Therapeutic communities were founded on the relational principles of belonging, safety, openness, inclusion, and empowerment, and Haigh (2013) argues that it is these same qualities of the environment that are seriously disrupted when a child is deprived, traumatised, or suffers significant loss. Therefore, the therapeutic community can act as a:

> a psychic space in which the things that went wrong or got stuck in primary emotional development can be re-experienced and re-worked in this artificially created setting. It might never have quite the impact as it could in childhood, but the experience can at least make a difference to expectations of relationships and the way in which care is sought of others thereafter. (Haigh, 2013, p. 14)

Whilst therapeutic communities in their pure sense have not become mainstream in the UK, ('TC proper'; Clark, 1965), the ideas that underpin them have been translated and adapted for use within more mainstream psychiatric practice (the 'therapeutic communities milieu approach') both historically, and more recently (Johnson & Haigh,

2010). Therapeutic communities currently exist in the UK for people diagnosed with 'personality disorders', psychoses, addictions, as well as for children and people with learning disabilities. From this praxis, the Royal College of Psychiatrists created the 'Enabling Environments' (EE) initiative (2010) and Psychologically-Informed Environments (Johnson & Haigh, 2010) to develop relational principles that could be used in general public health settings (e.g. a housing estate) and focused settings (e.g. a homeless hostel, acute ward, or prison wing).

There are also some residential settings that share the same relational values and principles to therapeutic communities. Soteria homes offer an alternative to hospitalisation for people with acute mental health needs, usually related to psychosis. The Soteria model was developed in California in the 1970s by psychiatrist Loren Mosher. The approach has been influential internationally and more recently, was recommended by the United Nations (UN Human Rights Council, 2017). The settings are homes, with small groups and open communication, consensual treatment (not focused on medication) and opportunities for activities alongside others (Lichtenberg, 2017). Like any therapeutic community, the therapeutic potential is in the group itself, and Soteria has the relational notions of 'being-with' and 'doing-with' at its core. Evidence suggests that Soteria is a low-cost, effective alternative to traditional psychiatric hospital and antipsychotics (Bola & Mosher, 2003; Mosher, 1999). Other respite houses have also been shown to be personally and financially effective for supporting people in crisis. These include Parachute in New York (Bouchery et al., 2018) and Maytree in London, UK (Briggs et al., 2007). By using peer-support workers (Parachute) and volunteer befrienders (Maytree), both services emphasise the relational values of trust, openness and confidentiality, and de-emphasise traditional medical models. Soteria, Parachute, and Maytree houses all emphasise care as a human relational activity that takes place in a home-like setting. The NHS Long Term Plan (NHS, 2019) suggests that this type of model works, and along with crisis cafes and host family projects, the NHS is committed to working with the third sector to provide these alternatives.

Another explicitly relational approach that has had significant impact and international reach is Open Dialogue (Seikkula et al., 1996). This methodology was developed in the 1990s, in the Finnish mental health system as an alternative way to treat people in psychological crisis. Unlike therapeutic communities that create a new relational setting, Open Dialogue works directly with the person's pre-existing social network. Both Soteria and Open Dialogue approaches have been described as client-centred and humanistic and both de-emphasise medication (Hahn, 2019), however, Open Dialogue operates within mainstream psychiatry. Working transdiagnostically, staff, the person in crisis, and their social network come together to talk transparently about what is happening. They meet as soon as possible and then again as required, typically every day at first. The treatment team involves relevant staff (e.g. inpatient and outpatient, or multi-agency), and they continue working with the person and their network, regardless of whether or not they are admitted to hospital, or how long they remain with the service. The person's social network includes family members, and anyone else of significance to the person in crisis, including, for example, an employer, workmate, friend, or neighbour. Who joins the meetings depends on who knows and is concerned about the crisis, who is available, and who may be of help. The work of the meetings is to speak about and make sense of the 'problem'. Bringing the whole network together into the treatment process is paramount because "the problem becomes dis-solved only if all who have defined it as a problem no longer communicate it as such" (Seikkula & Arnkil, 2006, p. 55).

Treatment in this model is described as "joint wondering" (Seikkula & Arnkil, 2006, p. 61) and the aim of meetings is to facilitate shared decision making, open communication into dialogue (rather than monologue), and to take seriously the experiences of the person in crisis. Seikkula and colleagues acknowledge the challenge of dialogue in the context of heightened anxiety and trauma, but they argue that staff can model the capacity to survive crisis through their embodied presence. This and their willingness to talk through difficult things, can be enough to provide a scaffold for others in the network. Through dialogue, they suggest, a new shared language, and therefore a new community, can be built around the person in crisis. The approach has been extremely successful in Finland, reducing antipsychotic use, hospitalisation and relapse rates, and improving 'symptoms' and occupational outcomes (Seikkula et al., 2003). Since the 2010s, several NHS mental health trusts in

England have been developing and implementing a peer-supported open dialogue approach, in which the professionals include peer-support workers (Razzaque & Stockmann, 2016). Initial findings suggest that these are well received by the person in crisis, as well as their loved ones and that there were significant improvements in functioning and wellbeing (Kinane et al., 2022). A large randomised controlled trial is currently underway (Pilling et al., 2022).

Peer support is fundamental in other approaches that operate both inside and outside of statutory services. Peer support is the mutual help that comes from dialogue between people with shared experiences, for example, substance misuse, such as in twelve step groups, like Alcholics Anonymous (AA). However, this informal mutual care has evolved into an important part of third sector and statutory mental health systems via the role of 'peer support worker' (Shalaby & Agyapong, 2020). Peer-led approaches to mental health care developed out of the survivor/service-user movements (e.g. Chamberlin, 1978), but the incorporation of peer support workers within the mainstream psychiatric services has been more recent (see Repper & Carter, 2010). Evidence is somewhat mixed, but it suggests that peer support interventions within mainstream psychiatric care can improve psychosocial outcomes (White et al., 2020). However, the fundamental nature of peer-to-peer support, which is based on a premise of equality, changes once employment comes into the equation, although peer support workers do seem to successfully provide hope, empowerment and inclusion, in a way that non-peer staff struggle to do (Repper & Carter, 2010).

Peer-led support programmes also thrive outside of statutory services. One example is Hearing Voices Groups, a survivor-led movement originating in the 1990s in Holland. Hearing Voices groups are now widespread in the UK and elsewhere. They are peer-led support groups for anyone who hears voices and offer a safer and supportive relational space where people can prioritise phenomenological explorations and meaning-making of their experiences alongside others with similar experiences. Voice-hearers, and those experiencing psychosis more generally, are amongst some of the most socially-isolated people in society (Thornicroft et al., 2004) and evidence shows that attendees report positive emotional, social and clinical outcomes, and value the relational support, which they cannot find available elsewhere (Longden et al., 2018).

Relational interventions have not disappeared from the mental health care landscape, despite the push towards individualism and independence. These alternative, relational approaches run from mainstream (but originally radical) interventions such as peer support programmes, to less common models of care, like therapeutic communities, through to innovative approaches, like Open Dialogue, that are just beginning to be incorporated within statutory services. Interventions that make the move into the mainstream are shaped by those same individualising and cost-saving discourses and policies that we have described above. However, those that stay outside of statutory services also suffer from a lack of funding and, on the whole, remain on the periphery, accessed only by those with enough social capital, insight or support to find them.

Conclusions

In order to work clinically with people in mental health crises or experiencing distress, relational thinking is imperative. However, the adult mental health system that we have currently in the UK, is driven by ideologies that prioritise individualism and independence, and which see mental health as something that happens 'inside' an individual person, rather than between people. Given these discourses, it is not surprising then that loneliness has also become a policy priority.

In 2013, Stephen Priebe and colleagues argued for a new, social psychiatry. They noted that as community care became established, services that actually worked with the community reduced. More mental health services are located outside of hospitals and within communities, but:

> Few services actively work at increasing social cohesion and social capital in their community to improve the mental health of local individuals. In an increasingly fragmented society, work with the community would help patients establish and maintain relationships with relatives, friends and wider social networks. (Priebe et al., 2013, p. 320)

Ten years later, Dianna Rose and Nikolas Rose (2023) are still making that same argument that services are failing to truly grapple with the social aspects of mental health. They suggest that for psychiatry to embrace relational working requires "a radical reimagination of the role and responsibilities of the medically trained psychiatrist within and outside the clinical encounter" (Rose & Rose, 2023, p. 46). This radical overhaul may even need to extend to the whole welfare system: Hilary Cottam (2018) argues for a 'relational welfare' that prioritises relationships, collectivity, and shared endeavour.

The dramatic shift necessary to move from the neoliberal view of the autonomous individual and the prioritisation of market relationships (back) to interdependency and the value of relationships for their own sake takes time. Meanwhile, people and communities facing distress are still searching for meaningful support. Those populations and communities with sufficient social cohesion—small, local groups, who have the means to access resources—are self-organising to meet their needs. One example is within queer mental health, where local, grassroots movements are taking place as alternatives or supplements to mainstream mental health support. For example, in Brighton, a place known as the 'gay capital' of the UK, a local LGBTQIA+ pub community supported each other's emotional and mental wellbeing through radical informal mental health practice (Wilcox & Graber, 2022). Other subgroups from the queer communities in Brighton also meet informally and spontaneously across the city, in spaces and places that hold meaning for them. For example, the Radical Faeries, a community group of queer people with an interest in eco-spirituality, meet at a firepit in a council-run orchard, while others meet at the nudist beach (Wilcox & Graber, forthcoming). Examples like this are supported by positive changes in the way that mental health is understood by the general population, and provide a necessary stop-gap for people in distress that cannot access humane, caring mental health support via mainstream services.

This chapter has provided a brief and necessarily partial account of just some of the ways that relational thinking has been included within, and excluded from, contemporary clinical practice in adult mental health care. From the fundamental assumption that the therapeutic relationship heals to the more complex relational interventions and practices that exist at the margins of mainstream services, relational thinking still survives in clinical contexts, albeit in pretty barren soils at present.

References

Atkinson, P. (2023). It is time we stopped colluding. *British Journal of Psychotherapy, 29*(2), 373–379.

Beck, A. (1976). *Cognitive therapy and the emotional disorders*. International Universities Press.

Beck, J. S. (2020). *Cognitive behavior therapy: Basics and beyond*. Guilford Publications.

Boden-Stuart, Z. V., Larkin, M., & Harrop, C. (2021). Young adults' dynamic relationships with their families in earlypsychosis: Identifying relational strengths and supporting relational agency. *Psychology and Psychotherapy: Theory, Research and Practice, 94*(3), 646–666.

Bola, J. R., & Mosher, L. R. (2003). Treatment of acute psychosis without neuroleptics: Two-year outcomes from the Soteria project. *The Journal of Nervous and Mental Disease, 191*(4), 219–229.

Bouchery, E. E., Barna, M., Babalola, E., Friend, D., Brown, J. D., Blyler, C., & Ireys, H. T. (2018). The effectiveness of a peer-Staffed crisis respite program as an alternative to hospitalization. *Psychiatric Services (Washington, D.C.), 69*(10), 1069–1074. https://doi.org/10.1176/appi.ps.201700451

Bowden, G., Holttum, S., Shankar, R., Cooke, A., & Kinderman, P. (Eds.). (2020). *Understanding depression: Why adults experience depression and what can help*. British Psychological Society.

Bowlby, J. (2005). *A secure base: Clinical applications of attachment theory* (Vol. 393). Taylor & Francis.

Bracken, P., Thomas, P., Timimi, S., et al. (2012). Psychiatry beyond the current paradigm. *British Journal of Psychiatry, 201*, 430–434.

Briggs, S., Webb, L., Buhagiar, J., & Braun, G. (2007). Maytree: A respite center for the suicidal: An evaluation. *Crisis, 28*(3), 140–147.

Calvert, R., & Kellett, S. (2014). Cognitive analytic therapy: A review of the outcome evidence base for treatment. *Psychology and Psychotherapy: Theory, Research and Practice, 87*(3), 253–277.

Care Quality Commission. (2022). *Monitoring the Mental Health Act in 2021/2022*. Care Quality Commission.

Chamberlin, J. (1978). *On our own: Patient-controlled alternatives to the mental health system*. McGraw-Hill.

Clark, D. H. (1965). The therapeutic community—Concept, practice and future. *The British Journal of Psychiatry, 111*(479), 947–949.

Cooke, A. (Ed.). (2017). *Understanding psychosis and schizophrenia* (Revised). British Psychological Society.

Cottam, H. (2018). *Radical help: How we can remake the relationships between us and revolutionise the welfare state*. Hachette.

Ebrahim, S., & Wilkinson, L. (2021). *Psychological services within the Acute Adult Mental Health Care Pathway Guidelines for service providers, policy makers and decision makers*. British Psychological Society.

Fairbairn, W. R. D. (1952). *An object-relations theory of the personality*. Basic Books.

Felitti, V. J., Anda, R. F., Nordenberg, D., Williamson, D. F., Spitz, A. M., Edwards, V., & Marks, J. S. (1998). Relationship of childhood abuse and household dysfunction to many of the leading causes of death in adults: The Adverse Childhood Experiences (ACE) study. *American Journal of Preventive Medicine, 14*(4), 245–258.

Firn, M. (2007). Assertive outreach: Has the tide turned against the approach? *Mental Health Practice, 10*(7), 24.

Firn, M., Hindhaugh, K., Hubbeling, D., Davies, G., Jones, B., & White, S. J. (2013). A dismantling study of assertive outreach services: Comparing activity and outcomes following replacement with the FACT model. *Social Psychiatry and Psychiatric Epidemiology, 48*, 997–1003.

Fonagy, P., et al. (2020). Dynamic interpersonal therapy for moderate to severe depression: A pilot randomized controlled and feasibility trial. *Psychological Medicine, 50*, 1010–1019. https://doi.org/10.1017/S0033291719000928

Gomez, L. (1997). *An introduction to object relations theory*. Free Association Press.

Hahn, P. D. (2019). Soteria house and open dialogue therapy. In P. D. Hahn (Ed.), *Madness and genetic determinism: Is mental illness in our genes?* (pp. 149–154). Palgrave Macmillan.

Haigh, R. (2013). The quintessence of a therapeutic environment. *Therapeutic Communities: The International Journal of Therapeutic Communities, 34*(1), 6–15.

Haigh, R. (2017). Therapeutic communities enter the world of evidence-based practice. *The British Journal of Psychiatry, 210*(5), 313–314.

Hannan, R. (2013). The Triangle of Care: carers included. *Journal of Public Mental Health, 12*(3), 171–172. https://doi.org/10.1108/JPMH-06-2013-0042

Hinshelwood, R., & Skogstad, W. (2000). *Observing organisations: Anxiety, defence and culture in health care*. Routledge.

Johnson, R., & Haigh, R. (2010). Social psychiatry and social policy for the 21st century-new concepts for new needs: The 'psychologically-informed environment'. *Mental Health and Social Inclusion, 14*(4), 30–35.

Johnstone, L., & Boyle, M., with Cromby, J., Dillon, J., Harper, D., Kinderman, P., Longden, E., Pilgrim, D., & Read, J. (2018). *The power threat meaning framework: Towards the identification of patterns in emotional distress, unusual experiences and troubled or troubling behaviour, as an alternative to functional psychiatric diagnosis*. British Psychological Society.

Jones, M. (1968). *Social psychiatry in practice*. Penguin.

Kinane, C., Osborne, J., Ishaq, Y., Colman, M., & MacInnes, D. (2022). Peer supported Open Dialogue in the National Health Service: Implementing and evaluating a new approach to Mental Health Care. *BMC Psychiatry, 22*(1), 138.

Klerman, G. L., & Weissman, M. M. (1994). *Interpersonal psychotherapy of depression: A brief, focused, specific strategy*. Jason Aronson.

Lemma, A., Target, M., & Fonagy, P. (2011). *Brief dynamic interpersonal therapy: A clinician's guide*. Oxford University Press.

Lichtenberg, P. (2017). From the closed ward to Soteria: A professional and personal journey. *Psychosis, 9*(4), 369–375.

Long, J., Ohlsen, S., Senek, M., Booth, A., Weich, S., & Wood, E. (2023). Realist synthesis of factors affecting retention of staff in UK adult mental health services. *BMJ Open, 13*(5), e070953.

Longden, E., Read, J., & Dillon, J. (2018). Assessing the impact and effectiveness of hearing voices network self-help groups. *Community Mental Health Journal, 54*, 184–188.

Main, T. (1946). The hospital as a therapeutic institution. *Bulletin of the Meninger Clinic, 10*, 66–70.

Marshall, M., & Lockwood, A. (1998). Assertive community treatment for people with severe mental disorders. *Cochrane Database of Systematic Reviews*. Issue 2. Art. No.: CD001089.

Mersey Care NHS Foundation Trust. (2019). *eRISK—My safety plan intervention resources pack: Safety planning intervention guide for 'significant other'*. Available at: https://www.merseycare.nhs.uk/application/files/3516/

2435/9120/Safety_planning_guide_for_significant_other.pdf. Retrieved 31 May 2023.
Morris, K., Hughes, N., Clarke, H., Tew, J., Mason, P., Galvani, S., Lewis, A., Loveless, L., Becker, S., & Burford, G. (2008). *Think family: A literature review of whole family approaches*. Cabinet Office.
Mosher, L. R. (1999). Soteria and other alternatives to acute psychiatric hospitalization: A personal and professional review. *The Journal of Nervous and Mental Disease, 187*(3), 142–149.
Moth, R. (2020). 'The business end': Neoliberal policy reforms and biomedical residualism in frontline community mental health practice in England. *Competition & Change, 24*(2), 133–153.
NHS. (2019). *The NHS long term plan*. Version 1.2. Available from: https://www.longtermplan.nhs.uk/wp-content/uploads/2019/08/nhs-long-term-plan-version-1.2.pdf. Retrieved 31 May 2023.
NICE. (2022). *Suicide prevention*. Quality standard QS189: Quality statement 4 Involving family, carers or friends. Available from: https://www.nice.org.uk/guidance/qs189/resources/suicide-prevention-pdf-75545729771461. Retrieved 31 May 2023.
NICE. (2023). *Self-harm: Assessment, management and preventing recurrence*. NICE guideline NG225. 1.4 Involving family members and carers. Available from: https://www.nice.org.uk/guidance/ng225/chapter/Recommendations#involving-family-members-and-carers. Retrieved 31 May 2023.
Norcross, J. C. (2019). *Psychotherapy relationships that work: Evidence-based responsiveness* (3rd ed.). Oxford University Press.
Norcross, J. C., & Wampold, B. E. (2011). Evidence-based therapy relationships: Research conclusions and clinical practices. *Psychotherapy (Chicago), 48*(1), 98–102. https://doi.org/10.1037/a0022161
Oxford Health NHS Foundation Trust. (2018). *Safety planning guidance*. Available at: https://www.rcpsych.ac.uk/docs/default-source/improving-care/nccmh/suicide-prevention/monthly-clinic/ohft-safety-planning-guidance.pdf. Retrieved 31 May 2023.
Pearce, S., & Haigh, R. (2017). Milieu approaches and other adaptations of therapeutic community method: Past and future. *Therapeutic Communities: The International Journal of Therapeutic Communities, 38*(3), 136–146.
Pilling, S., Clarke, K., Parker, G., James, K., Landau, S., Weaver, T., Razzaque, R., & Craig, T. (2022). Open dialogue compared to treatment as usual for adults experiencing a mental health crisis: Protocol for the ODDESSI multi-

site cluster randomised controlled trial. *Contemporary Clinical Trials, 113*, 106664.
Pinquart, M., Oslejsek, B., & Teubert, D. (2016). Efficacy of systemic therapy on adults with mental disorders: A meta-analysis. *Psychotherapy Research, 26*(2), 241–257.
Priebe, S., Burns, T., & Craig, T. K. J. (2013). The future of academic psychiatry may be social. *British Journal of Psychiatry, 202*, 319–320.
Rappoport, R. (1960). *Community as doctor*. Tavistock.
Razzaque, R., & Stockmann, T. (2016). An introduction to peer-supported open dialogue in mental healthcare. *BJPsych Advances, 22*(5), 348–356.
Read, J., Perry, B. D., Moskowitz, A., & Connolly, J. (2001). The contribution of early traumatic events to schizophrenia in some patients: A traumagenic neurodevelopmental model. *Psychiatry, 64*(4), 319–345.
Read, J., Fosse, R., Moskowitz, A., & Perry, B. (2014). The traumagenic neurodevelopmental model of psychosis revisited. *Neuropsychiatry, 4*(1), 65–79.
Repper, J., & Carter, T. (2010). *Using personal experience to support others with similar difficulties: A review of the literature on peer support in mental health services*. Together/University of Nottingham/NSUN. Available from: www.together-uk.org/wpcontent/uploads/downloads/2011/11/usingpersexperience.pdf. Retrieved 31 May 2023.
Rizq, R. (2012). The perversion of care: Psychological therapies in a time of IAPT. *Psychodynamic Practice, 18*(1), 7–24.
Rizq, R., & Jackson, C. (2019). *The industrialisation of care: Counselling, psychotherapy and the impact of IAPT*. PCCS Books.
Rogers, C. R. (1951). *Client-centred therapy; its current practice, implications, and theory*. Houghton Mifflin.
Rose, D., & Rose, N. (2023). Is 'another' psychiatry possible? *Psychological Medicine, 53*, 46–54.
Royal College of Psychiatrists. (2010). *Enabling environments* [online]. Available from: http://www.rcpsych.ac.uk/quality/quality,accreditationaudit/enablingenvironments.aspx. Accessed Jan 2011.
Ryle, A., & Kerr, I. (2020). *Introducing cognitive analytic therapy: Principles and practice of a relational approach to mental Health*. Wiley.
Ryle, A., Leighton, T., & Pollock, P. (1997). *Cognitive analytic therapy and borderline personality disorder: The model and the method*. John Wiley & Sons Inc.
Sadusky, A. & Spinks, J. (2022). Psychologists' engagement in reflective practice and experiences of burnout: A correlational analysis. *Reflective Practice International and Multidisciplinary Perspectives, 23*(5).

Samaritans. (n.d.). *Supporting someone with suicidal thoughts: 3. Creating a safety plan*. Available at: https://www.samaritans.org/how-we-can-help/if-youre-worried-about-someone-else/supporting-someone-suicidal-thoughts/creating-safety-plan/ Retrieved 31 May 2023.

Seikkula, J., & Arnkil, T. E. (2006). *Dialogical meetings in social networks*. Routledge.

Seikkula, J., Aaltonen, J., & Alakare, B. (1996). Treating psychosis in Western Lapland: Reflective processes and open dialogue instead of hospitalization and heavy medication. *ISM Skriftserie, 35*, 156–171.

Seikkula, J., Alakare, B., Aaltonen, J., Holma, J., Rasinkangas, A., & Lehtinen, V. (2003). Open dialogue approach: Treatment principles and preliminary results of a two-year follow-up on first episode schizophrenia. *Ethical Human Sciences and Services, 5*(3), 163–182.

Shalaby, R. A. H., & Agyapong, V. I. (2020). Peer support in mental health: Literature review. *JMIR Mental Health, 7*(6), e15572.

Sheffler, J. L., Stanley, I., & Sachs-Ericsson, N. (2020). ACEs and mental health outcomes. In G. Asmundson & T. Afifi (Eds.), *Adverse childhood experiences: Using evidence to advance research, practice, policy, and prevention* (pp. 47–69). Academic.

Stanbridge, R., & Burbach, F. (2007). Developing family-inclusive mainstream mental health services. *Journal of Family Therapy, 29*(1), 21–43.

Stanley, B. & Brown, G. K., with Karlin, B., Kemp, J. E., & VonBergen, H. A. (2008). Safety plan treatment manual to reduce suicide risk: Veteran version. : United States Department of Veterans Affairs, 12.

Taylor, B. (2015). *The last asylum: A memoir of madness in our times*. Hamish Hamilton.

Tew, J., Ramon, S., Slade, M., Bird, V., Melton, J., & Le Boutillier, C. (2012). Social factors and recovery from mental health difficulties: A review of the evidence. *The British Journal of Social Work, 42*(3), 443–460.

Tew, J., Morris, K., White, S., Featherstone, B., & Fenton, S. J. (2015). What has happened to 'Think Family'—Challenges and achievements in implementing family inclusive practice. *Pavilion Annual Parental Mental Health and Child Welfare Work, 1*, 59–64.

Thornicroft, G., Tansella, M., Becker, T., Knapp, M., Leese, M., Schene, A., Vazquez-Barquero, J. L., & the EPSILON Study Group. (2004). The personal impact of schizophrenia in Europe. *Schizophrenia Research, 69*(2–3), 125–132.

Topping, S., & Gamble, C. (n.d.). *PNAs and reflective practice in mental health services.* Available at: https://www.england.nhs.uk/nursingmidwifery/delivering-the-nhs-ltp/professional-nurse-advocate/case-studies/pnas-and-reflective-practice-in-mental-health-services/. Accessed 31 May 2023.

Tyrer, P. (2000). Are small case-loads beautiful in severe mental illness? *British Journal of Psychiatry, 177*, 386–387.

UNISON. (2017). *Struggling to cope: Mental health staff and services under pressure*. UNISON.

von Sydow, K., Beher, S., Schweitzer, J., & Retzlaff, R. (2010). The efficacy of systemic therapy with adult patients: A meta-content analysis of 38 randomized controlled trials. *Family Process, 49*(4), 457–485.

Waft, Y. (2011). Is CAT in danger of being squeezed out of the NHS? *Reformulation*, Summer, 18–21.

White, S., Foster, R., Marks, J., Morshead, R., Goldsmith, L., Barlow, S., Sin, J., & Gillard, S. (2020). The effectiveness of one-to-one peer support in mental health services: A systematic review and meta-analysis. *BMC Psychiatry, 20*(1), 1–20.

Wilcox, C., & Graber, R. (2022). 'We the Marlborough': Elucidating Users' Experience of Radical, Informal Therapeutic Practices Within a Queer Community Pub. In *The Palgrave Handbook of Innovative Community and Clinical Psychologies* (pp. 201–222). Cham: Springer International Publishing.

Winnicott, D. W. (1958). *Collected papers: Through paediatrics to psycho-analysis*. Tavistock Publications.

Part II

Relational Trauma; Relational Recovery

4

Family Relatedness for Māori Survivors of Familial Childhood Sexual Abuse

Nicola Harrison and Jade Le Grice

Childhood sexual abuse (CSA) has significant impacts for the affected individual. Familial childhood sexual abuse (FCSA) impacts the whole family. When offender and victim are located within the family, the complexity of relational impacts augment quickly. Every member of a family has their own set of relationships to re-examine after a disclosure of FCSA within the group. Multi-relationality and the pronounced divergence in lived experience can make the journey from distress to recovery particularly relationally fraught for survivors of FCSA and their families.

CSA is recognised as a significant international social problem. Global prevalence rates suggest that 27–36% of girls and 13–16% of boys are victims of CSA (Fanslow et al., 2007; Yancey & Hansen, 2010). In Indigenous communities, the incidence rate is in orders of higher magnitude. Amongst Indigenous communities in Canada, women are three times more likely to experience sexual assault (Du Mont et al., 2017).

N. Harrison (✉) • J. Le Grice
Psychology and Sociology, The University of Auckland,
Auckland, New Zealand
e-mail: n.harrison@auckland.ac.nz

Z. Boden-Stuart, M. Larkin (eds.), *Relationships and Mental Health*,
https://doi.org/10.1007/978-3-031-50047-3_4

Indigenous children in Australia are two–four times more likely to be victims of CSA (Australian Institute of Health and Welfare, 2014), and Māori children in Aotearoa (New Zealand) are twice as likely to be victims of CSA than non-Māori (Fanslow et al., 2007; Mayhew & Reilly, 2006). Of all these victims, 90% know their abuser, and over a quarter (26%) of perpetrators are family members (HELP, 2022; Ministry of Justice, 2022).

Moving from distress to recovery after FCSA is always relationally complex. It can be even more so for Indigenous survivors due, in part, to the bearing that connectedness with one's family has on one's individual identity and the ongoing impacts of colonisation. This chapter explores how Māori survivors of FCSA are leaning on Indigenous ways of being and doing family to support this journey and then are passing the benefits on to the next generation.

Whanaungatanga and Doing Family

To understand how FCSA affects the experience of family and relatedness for Māori survivors, we first need to lay a foundation of how Māori understand family and experience familial connectedness. Whānau is commonly translated into English as 'family' or 'extended family' (Pihama & Lee-Morgan, 2022). It is a social unit within Māori society that typically consists of three or four generations of family living in close proximity and undertaking shared activities for the provision and prosperity of the collective group (Pere, 1982; Walker, 2004). The distinction between family and whānau is an important one. From what we can learn about pre-settler Māori society, we know whānau were sources of knowledge, learning, history, love, care, protection, strength and social control. These functions were designed to be delivered by the multi-generational structure of whānau. Grandparents taught stories and social norms to young children while parents undertook the physical labour required to feed and protect the whānau (Pere, 1982; Walker, 2004). Colonisation nuclearised whānau into families, splitting whānau into smaller, more dislocated[1] units. The immediate effect was that the multi-generational structure upon which the systems of order and knowledge transmission relied was severed.

Whanaungatanga cannot be concretely defined. Despite countless Māori writers' theorising, discussing and conceptualising, there remains no standardised definition. However, for our purposes, whanaungatanga can be thought of as the ways in which Māori *do* family. Western theorists have come to think of family, in the last 20 years or so, in similar ways as Māori scholars have described whanaungatanga. Māori scholar, Rose Pere (1982), described whanaungatanga as a system of practices rooted in mutual commitment that strengthens kinship ties. Well-known English sociologist David H J Morgan (2011a, b) described family as something that is achieved through the active *doing* of regular, everyday practices. Morgan posits that participating in family practices is how meaning is given to the relationships of those involved (Morgan, 2011a). Examples of such practices can include food/feeding practices, practices of care and practices of familial narrative creation (and reproduction). These same practices could also be categorised according to the overarching principles of whanaungatanga: wairuatanga (spirituality),[2] manaakitanga (hospitality, reciprocity, caring and role responsibility), kotahitanga (collectivity and unity), mana motuhake (self-determination), kaitiakitanga (to lead and guide) and tiakitanga (unconditional love and commitment) (Le Grice et al., 2017; McNatty & Roa, 2002; Ritchie, 1992; Sharman, 2019). Food/feeding practices and practices of care could, quite comfortably, be understood as expressions of manaakitanga (hospitality and caring). Familial narrative creation and reproduction could seem harder to align at first conceptually. Yet, Carol Smart (2007) asserts that stories and histories are part of what binds us together as families. Thus, we can see that the telling and re-telling of stories can be seen as an enactment of kotahitanga as the practice creates collectivity and unity. These are but two examples of how modern sociological thinking about

[1] Policy and legislation meant Māori were moved from living on their own land in whānau into cities as nuclear families. Māori were thus social and economically dislocated.

[2] These bracketed translations are exceptionally reductive and have been used in this way purely for the purpose of communicating a very basic understanding of these concepts upon which further discussion can be based.

families can be seen as sitting parallel, in some ways, to whanaungatanga or how whānau *do* family. For Māori,[3] relationality is at the heart of whanaungatanga (Le Grice et al., 2017). It provides the basis for relatedness within and without whānau boundaries (Durie, 2011).

Whanaungatanga is one of the constructs that sits at the heart of whānau; another is whakapapa. Whakapapa is most commonly translated as meaning 'genealogy'. However, in its most complete form, whakapapa is the scaffold by which all things are connected (Barlow, 1991). Whakapapa is the method by which the knowledge of the world is held together (Tau, 2001). This ontological perspective is crucial to understanding the impact of FCSA for Māori survivors and their whānau. Whakapapa connects us with our tīpuna (ancestors), our tamariki (children) and the world around us. For many Māori, whakapapa means that one is the embodiment of their history personified in present time (Webb & Shaw, 2011).

Furthermore, the actions of individuals contribute to the legacy that will be passed on to future generations (Webb & Shaw, 2011). This means, in te ao Māori (the Māori world), the actions of each individual impact the collective (Mikaere, 1994). A potentially parallel perspective to this concept is presented by Carol Smart (2007). Smart describes such a condition as "being embedded in a family history" (Smart, 2007, p. 81). However, unlike whakapapa in te ao Māori, the self as embedded in family history can often go unremarked in Western families (Smart, 2007) and is often viewed as optional (Elizabeth, 2019).

Practices which are faithful to the principles of whanaungatanga assume respect of whakapapa; they show respect to the belief that one's actions are intimately interwoven with their family; past, present and future (Rameka, 2016). Actions such as abuse are not in keeping with whanaungatanga. Abuse has no respect for whakapapa. Abuse inflicted upon any member of a whānau is violence against the whole whakapapa line (Mikaere, 1994; Pihama et al., 2016). Thus, the fallout of FCSA is detrimental to those living in present time and the entire whakapapa. As

[3] Māori are not a homogeneous collective. Iwi (tribes) vary significantly across Aotearoa (NZ) and I cannot presume to speak for all people.

both victim and perpetrator exist within the same whakapapa, the effects of FCSA are twice amplified.

Here we come up against one of the central paradoxes of dealing with FCSA within whānau. How does one navigate relatedness, within a paradigm of absolute connectedness, given the antithetical context of FCSA? This question is answered unambiguously by the kaiāwhina (contributors) to this research. They navigate the complex processes of managing distress and seeking recovery, for themselves and their whānau, by leaning on whanaungatanga.

Kaupapa Māori Methodology

Kaupapa Māori methodology developed within a broader research context where historical and contemporary research accepted racist, imperialist, and culturally appropriated interpretations of Māori lives and worldviews as knowledge about Māori (Bishop, 1999; Mikaere, 2011). Historically, much research defined Māori as 'other' and different from dominant Western culture (Smith, 2000, 2012; Tuhiwai Smith, 2012). Kaupapa Māori research situates Māori views of the world as the norm, subverting the dynamics that have marginalised us in research (Moewaka Barnes, 2000). Small but significant details demonstrate the decision to emphasise Māori epistemologies (Tuhiwai Smith, 2012). For example, participants in this research are known as kaiāwhina, meaning contributors. The term kaiāwhina is used rather than participant or respondent as it acknowledges the collaborative process of knowledge creation undertaken in this research. It acknowledges that the shared stories are a gift given to this work by those with the horrible privilege of holding them.

Furthermore, it acknowledges that those who are contributing their stories and the researcher who collects and makes meaning from them are equally necessary in the research process. Another example of terminology use, particularly in the analysis phase, is the application of the term whanaungatanga. Many kaiāwhina shared how perpetrators often manipulated whanaungatanga principles to oppress, isolate and abuse family members. To differentiate between actions that manipulate whanaunga tanga principles to achieve oppressive ends and enactments of whanaungatanga that strengthen and empower, I have adopted a linguistic technique of te ao Māori and modified the term whanaungatanga. Whanaungatanga hē[4] describes enactments that may be called whanaungatanga but are, in reality, contrary to tikanga Māori (protocols, correct way of doing things, boundaries) and are more reflective of coloniser ideology than tikanga. This is distinct from whanaungatanga iho,[5] which are enactments in keeping with the love, care, commitment and respect of whakapapa that is characteristic of whanaungatanga principles. Whanaungatanga, in its fullest expression, has the potential to foster the well-being of people (Hamley et al., 2021; Le Grice, 2019). Whanaungatanga iho are practices that reflect ancestral principles of whanaungatanga without manipulation and fulfil the promise of fostering well-being.

Kaupapa Māori methodology drove the incorporation of consultation, cognisance to the importance of kanohi ki te kanohi (face to face) interactions and the use of pūrākau (story/narrative) analysis. From the outset of this research, a vital support team member has been a Kaitiaki (one who leads and guides). This role brings mātauranga Māori (Māori knowledge) to the project that is able to validate assertions of whanaungatanga, whānau and other tikanga Māori. In addition, along this research journey, members of various Māori communities have been consulted. Many of the opportunities for consultation were created through the third-party recruitment process.

A third-party recruitment method was used to assist in safe kaiāwhina selection. The principle investigator met kanohi ki te kanohi with counsellors who work with Māori survivors of FCSA. In these meetings, they could get to know her, her intentions in pursuing this work and her way

[4] Hē, when used as a modifier, translates in English as incorrectly, in the wrong way and indicates something done or handled incorrectly. Moorfield, J. C. (2022a). *Te Aka: Māori Dictionary, Hē.* https://maoridictionary.co.nz/search?idiom=&phrase=&proverb=&loan=&histLoanWords=&keywords=-he

[5] Iho has two translations in English: the middle portion of the umbilical cord; and the essence or the heart of something (Moorfield, J. C. (2022b). *Te Aka: Māori Dictionary, Iho*. https://maoridictionary.co.nz/search?idiom=&phrase=&proverb=&loan=&histLoanWords=&keywords=iho.) Iho is similarly used elsewhere in te reo Māori (Māori language) such as toi iho which is "the unique registered Aotearoa New Zealand trademark of Maori quality and authenticity" (Toi Iho. (2022). *About Toi Iho*. Retrieved 24/7/22 from http://www.toiiho.co.nz/about-toi-iho/).

of being. This element of project design addresses the spiritual element of connecting with someone. We were asking counsellors to put us in contact with their clients; thus, they needed to be able to share space with the principle investigator and sense my wairua.[6] This was a critical part of the project design, particularly given its sensitive nature.

Each counsellor received invitation packs to pass on to people they knew who met the study requirements, including the safety requirements. Each pack included all the information a potential kaiāwhina needed to know about contributing to the project. If someone chose to contribute, they contacted us directly. This method ensured a professional safety assessment was made of each potential contributor before an invitation to participate was extended.

One-on-one interviews also followed Kaupapa Māori protocols. This entailed the provision and consuming of kai (food), opening and closing with karakia (prayer),[7] a relaxed and respectful atmosphere, and the gifting of koha (a voluntary gift of thanks) to the kaiāwhina. Seventeen Māori survivors of FCSA were interviewed. Interviews took place in the kaiāwhina's town of residence, often in their home. These ranged from the Far North of Aotearoa to the Bay of Plenty, spanning approximately two-thirds of the North Island of Aotearoa. Their combined iwi (tribe) affiliations spanned Aotearoa. Kaiāwhina ranged from 36 to 68 years of age and predominantly identified as female; two of the sample identified as male, and one identified as two-spirit. All but one[8] of these 17

[6] Wairua is commonly translated as 'spirit'. The literal translation is 'two waters'. This refers to the combining of physical attributes – such as tone of voice, affect and body language – with spiritual attributes – such as the feeling you get in someone's presence, or a sense of safety or danger when someone speaks. As two waters join together, so do physical and spiritual attributes work in concert in wairua. To feel a person's wairua could be thought of as having an instinct about their character or a sixth sense. However, keep in mind that these are Western concepts that are not the same as wairua, but may help in understanding wairua.

[7] Where kaiāwhina wished to do so.

[8] One kaiāwhina was abused by a close family friend.

kaiāwhina were sexually abused[9] by at least one (in many cases multiple) close family member[10] before age 15.[11]

Analysis of interview transcripts was done using a bricolage approach. Bricolage, proposed by Lévi-Strauss, calls for the researcher (or the bricoleur) to employ a variety of knowledges from a broad base of experience (Lévi-Strauss, 1966). This approach opens space for Indigenous ontologies and epistemologies to be utilised and thus acknowledged as valid. This space has been named by Jenny Lee (2009) as that of the Indigenous bricoleur. An Indigenous bricolage approach is particularly useful where the 'data' being gathered is a complex network of lived experiences interpreted in an interplay between contributor and analyst (Lee, 2009). Part of the Indigenous epistemological approach to analysis is using pūrākau (stories/narratives) to gain insight into the underlying drivers and sentiments of the experiences shared by kaiāwhina. Pūrākau as a method of analysis is an extension of pūrākau as traditional forms of Māori narratives. Pūrākau contain "philosophical thought, epistemological constructs, cultural codes, and world views that are fundamental to our identity as Māori" (Lee, 2009, p. 1).

Survivor Experiences of Whanaungatanga

Let us be clear: the family of every person spoken with has been a site of traumatising abuse. Nevertheless, because whānau extend beyond the confines of nuclear families, they have also been able to provide experiences of whanaungatanga iho. In some cases, the whānau to whom survivors have turned have been families of choice; in others, it has been members of the community, teachers and counsellors, nephews, uncles

[9] Very broad definitions of sexual abuse are used across existing research, using terms such as "sexual activities" Draucker, C. B., & Martsolf, D. S. (2008). Storying Childhood Sexual Abuse. *Qualitative Health Research, 18*(8), 1034–1048. This includes activities such as viewing pornography, displaying of genitalia or watching masturbation. However, for this project sexual abuse is defined as sexual contact—one sided fondling of genitalia (perpetrator on survivor, survivor on perpetrator), mutual fondling of genitalia, penetration/rape and/or oral sex (perpetrator on survivor, survivor on perpetrator).

[10] As defined earlier: Parent, Grandparent, sibling, cousin, Aunt or Uncle

[11] This is the age used as a marker for the conclusion of 'childhood' in similar research.

and even partners of family members. Such networks of relatedness provided kaiāwhina with access to whanaungatanga iho, distinct from whanaungatanga hē, which, at best ignored and at worst, justified their abuse. Kaiāwhina could clearly distinguish between whanaungatanga iho—which they found to be a source of resilience and strength—and the oppressive and punitive whanaungatanga hē.

In the following sections, an amalgamated case study approach is used to facilitate a discussion of the research outcomes. The story of 'Kaitiana' is crafted from the experiences of different kaiāwhina across the sample and written from the perspective of the principle investigator who sat with her and received her story.

Whanaungatanga Iho Supports Movement Through Distress into Recovery

Kaitiana was abused by no less than five men in her family: a brother, some uncles, a cousin or two. And that's just the sexual abuse. Despite this, she sits before me at almost 60 years of age, a strong and determined woman. As a young child, her Nan would come and stay with her family. Kaitiana's Nan would sit on the floor with her, cooking or weaving, as she told her stories about their whakapapa. Kaitiana recalls with fondness how much her Nan adored her: "You knew that you were absolutely loved and adored. We're not talking words. It's by every action that she had."

When Kaitiana was ten, her Nan died. That was when everything changed. Kaitiana credits the experiences she shared with her Nan with giving her the resilience to survive abuse. "That first ten years was what got me through abuse. It was that whanaungatanga, that kaitiakitanga[12], that tikanga[13], manaakitanga...It was the foundation. The wairuatanga, the waiata[14], to get your feelings out and to be a Māori warrior princess...And, actually, I know if I hadn't had that first ten years, I would never have made it," she says, misty-eyed.

---

[12] Leading and guiding.

[13] Knowledge of boundaries and proper ways to do things.

[14] Songs.

Kaitiana identifies several aspects of whanaungatanga that she believes enabled her to survive abuse: kaitiakitanga (leading and guiding), tikanga (boundaries, protocols, proper way of doing things), manaakitanga (care, hospitality, role responsibility), wairuatanga (spirituality). She describes activities that we can identify as whanaungatanga iho. Cooking is an enactment of manaakitanga, teaching weaving is an enactment of kaitiakitanga and sharing stories of whakapapa fosters kotahitanga.

Kaitiana says that these experiences of whanaungatanga iho formed a 'foundation' for her. Her use of the word foundation evokes imagery of a grounded and stable sense of self in te ao Māori. Knowing tikanga gave her a solid understanding of boundaries and expectations of appropriateness. Experiencing manaakitanga gave her confidence in her value and how much she was loved. She even specifies that through waiata, she learnt how to express her feelings and 'be a Māori warrior princess'. The strength in a warrior and the royal value of a princess are the elements of self gifted to Kaitiana by her Nan through whanaungatanga iho.

Curious, I ask Kaitiana how whanaungatanga has helped her survive. She shares a story about how she communicates with her ancestors through wairuatanga: "Throughout my life, every time something's really bad, or I feel like I'm in a dark place, I will get my Nan [coming to me]…yeah, the main person that guides me is my Nan. There's been times where I have asked her to put me to sleep because I can't sleep. I haven't slept for days, and I just call out to her, 'Nan, help me. Help me sleep.' And, I'll be gone. And, then wake up the next day like, 'thank you'…I leaned on [my Nan]. That was my go-to, to take me away from what was happening in the real world, was the old people. Yeah. I talk to them, and yeah, it just really helped me get through because you were alone, and you think no one else knows what you're going through, you know?"

Accessing whanaungatanga iho through wairuatanga enabled Kaitiana to affect her external and internal environment. In Kaitiana's experience, her Nan affected her temporal state—by enabling her to get some much-needed rest—and her emotional and psychological state. Privileging a Māori ontological paradigm allows us to accept Kaitiana's experience of relatedness with her whakapapa beyond this life as valid. Wairuatanga provides access to power for otherwise powerless children. Most[15] of the kaiāwhina experienced feelings of power, strength, reassurance, love and guidance in communications with tīpuna through wairuatanga, despite the loneliness and neglect they felt in what Kaitiana calls 'the real world'.

Kaitiana's eyes twinkle; she is excited to share this next story. She recalls a time when she was struggling: "I was going through a difficult time...I was sort of questioning what my purpose was in all of this struggle and tension, I thought my [world] was going to come crumbling down and it was then, it was after that, that I saw myself in the mirror with a full face moko (whispers) which is a man. It was almost like a reminder of my strength... I remember thinking to myself, "I'm, as, I'm as strong as any man", you know, "don't let the bastard get you down". It was at that point I realised I wasn't alone and I sure as hell wasn't going to let another guy take me down." Kaitiana grins mischievously. I can tell it is an experience that has encouraged and emboldened her.

The imagery provided to Kaitiana through wairuatanga in this moment is a powerful message of solidarity, strength and a reminder of whakapapa. Being part of a chain in our whakapapa, we represent our whakapapa in the present time (Rameka, 2016). The appearance of a full-face moko (tattoo), which is worn by men, is a reminder that our connection with whakapapa is not bound by gender; we are an embodiment of all elements of our whakapapa. A moko can represent many different things. In the most general of senses, moko typically communicate identity and represent love, pain, learning, change and strength (Te Awekotuku, 2006). Such symbolism evokes thoughts of how transformation can take place through pain processing and foreshadows the permanent commitment to wellness and stopping abuse that Kaitiana has since demonstrated in her life.

Research on the impacts of CSA tends to paint a rather bleak prognosis for survivors: intimate partner violence, substance abuse and suicidal ideation. Every kaiāwhina to this project experienced some combination of these expected outcomes. However, those survivors who have

[15] 11 out of 16.

whanaungatanga iho on which to lean have sources of reassurance, comfort and purpose that can be brought to bear in the daily combat of destructive influences.

Enacting Whanaungatanga Iho to Create Long-Lasting Change

Kaitiana spent her adult life helping others. She graduated from university and dedicated herself to a profession where she was able to help whānau with their trauma. Yet, Kaitiana wanted to create change in her whānau too. "I saw two generations or three generations of kids in my time working…I can't change [the abuse] that happened, but what I can do is help make sure that you know and your family knows that it is not to continue. And, to normalise talking about [abuse that occurs], what I realised I would have to do, was to stop the abuse in the generations. I'm a nanny and a grandmother, a great aunty, and a great-great aunty…It cannot be normal, and it cannot continue."

Intergenerational sexual violence is just that, intergenerational. It stands to reason that combating it will also be an intergenerational project. Every kaiāwhina who shared their story with me wanted to create change in their whānau. Despite having differing levels of contact and intimacy with their immediate family, all kaiāwhina shared the same desire to create better conditions for their nieces and nephews, their children and grandchildren. One way they are doing this is by creating spaces for conversations about sexual violence and sexual safety. Part of what has allowed FCSA to continue has been the reluctance, fear and shame associated with speaking up and disclosing to whānau. Some whānau did not talk about sexuality, let alone sexual abuse. Others would liken anyone who spoke about abuse to fruit that had gone off, labelling them 'crazy' or 'bad'.

The fear and shame of disclosing sexual abuse are well documented. However, the sociohistorical context of colonised Aotearoa means there are additional layers of reluctance for Māori to disclose abuse within whānau. Māori are over-represented at every stage of the justice system (Ministry of Justice, 2021), whanaungatanga continues to be portrayed as a source of familial dysfunction (Le Grice et al., 2017), and of all the children uplifted by the state in Aotearoa, 69% of them are Māori (Office of the Children's Commissioner, 2020). There is justifiable apprehension about governmental intervention in Māori communities. Thus, to disclose abuse and take action against a member of the whānau is often perceived as going against tikanga Māori and doing things 'the Pākehā way' or the colonised way. Creating long-lasting change by speaking up about abuse is a slow process. Often whānau members can feel that to keep quiet about abuse is tikanga. This is a fallacy. It is whanaungatanga hē. Silence about sexual violence does not reflect the principles of our tīpuna who treasured children as precious gifts. That is tikanga. Children are the future of the whakapapa and are to be valued as such (Taonui, 2010). It is centuries of embedded colonised attitudes that has created a space where resistance continues within whānau to naming abusers and dealing with them openly.[16] It is slow, but change is happening.

Kaitiana tells me about how she began to have open and clear conversations with the children in her whānau about what was appropriate and inappropriate physical interaction. To her surprise, she found that opening spaces for discussion meant that the adults in her whānau began slowly opening up too. She recalls, "but, then, what was wonderful is the parents would start asking questions. Like, I remember my brother coming to me, and he goes, 'So Sis, when do we start talking to the kids?' Because they'd see me doing it and how engaged the kids were."

Unfortunately, not all Kaitiana's siblings accepted her openness about FCSA. Some of her whānau considered her and her family "the bad ones" and would keep her separated from her nieces and nephews. But, the next generation knew that Kaitiana was the one to come to when they needed support. One niece in particular, who had a baby herself and had been raised by her grandmother, was turned away by the rest of the whānau when her grandmother died. It was Kaitiana that this niece turned to for

[16] As recently as the 1940s, where abuse was discovered between members of a whānau, the offender could be sent away or removed from the home (Metge, 1995). Before settler contact, an offender could be ordered to die or slaved out to another iwi (Pere, 1982; Sharman, 2019). Either way, while an offender could not be removed from whakapapa, they were diminished to a point of almost non-existence (Metge, 1995; Pere, 1982). They would lose their authority and status and their name would not be mentioned (Metge, 1995).

refuge. In Kaitiana's words, "she [my niece] told the police that I was probably the only one that would give her a chance." Her niece was right; Kaitiana took her in. She continues the story, "we picked her [my niece] up, and she was so scared that day, and she cried, and we just laughed and made a joke of it, you know, 'phewf, now you're the bad one too eh, looks like you came to the right place'." Kaitiana and I laugh. We laugh from the belly, the kind of laugh characteristic of Māori; big and loud, right from the soul.

And why does Kaitiana continue to help and support a group of people who characterise her negatively? Her little ones used to ask her the same thing: "[when my kids were younger, they would] often say, 'why do you help them? Why do you?'. [I answer,] because that is us, that's who *we* are."

In examining the experiences of incremental change shared by kaiāwhina, a well-known Māori symbol came to mind; the koru. A koru is representative of a new, unfurling silver fern frond. It represents new life and growth. Each kaiāwhina started their project of change as a single individual. Yet, as they continue to practise whanaungatanga iho, those around them experience the effects of their enactments. Several kaiāwhina shared how, one by one, members of their whānau are starting to speak out. People are slowly following their example and are joining them in refusing to accept whanaungatanga hē. As they disclose their experiences and speak out about FCSA in their whānau, survivors are transitioning into kaitiaki. They stand proudly as a voice for change, even against the many voices that tell them they are 'bad' or 'crazy'. They are taking their experiences of whanaungatanga iho and passing on the ability to trust in te ao Māori as a source of strength and resilience to the next generation. Through the example of survivors and their enactments of whanaungatanga iho, we can hold hope for a safer, healthier future for our children.

Conclusion

Childhood sexual abuse is unacceptable; its prevalence within Indigenous communities is even more so. Colonising discourse continues to vilify Indigenous ways of being and doing in settler societies despite consonances between UK and US sociological theories of family practices with whanaungatanga principles as creating belonging, intimacy and meaningful identity. The ongoing project of colonisation[17] disconnected many Indigenous peoples from the multi-generational social structure which would have passed down knowledge of tikanga, leaving generations of Māori to re-construct an understanding of whanaungatanga from the resources available. The resultant can be whanaungatanga hē; enactments of whanaungatanga that are either purposefully harmful or, more commonly, newer instantiations formed in the context of the colonisation but attached to Māori terminology. This research shows whanaungatanga hē as distinct from whanaungatanga iho through which, even in arguably the worst of circumstances, te ao Māori can be a source of strength and resilience. While whanaungatanga hē often upholds intergenerational abuse and familial dysfunction, whanaungatanga iho could be the antidote. Māori survivors of FCSA are utilising the strength and resilience they find in whanaungatanga iho and te ao Māori to manage their environments, navigate their relationships with whānau and hold firm in their resolve to stop FCSA from continuing into the next generation.

The paradigm of whakapapa means that we are responsible to those who come after us. Kaitiana—as a representation of this sample of survivors—stands firmly in her belief of what she can do; raise her voice.

> *I can't stay quiet. I'm never going to be quiet. While there's still breath in me, I will share my story on behalf of the voiceless. If I can just change one person's life, open one more person's eyes, open one more person's heart. I'll never, till the day I die, keep the conspiracy of silence because it does not keep people safe, it cannot be normal, and it cannot continue.* (Combined quote from three kaiāwhina)

[17] This could manifest as adoption of colonising social discourse and practice, such as heteropatriarchal norms of male dominance over women and children, or as a response to coloniser hostility, such as hesitancy to seek aid from governmental agencies for fear of the punitive effects of systemic racism.

Glossary

Please note these translations are exceptionally reductive and are only intended to provide a general understanding of te reo (Māori language) as used in this chapter to assist in accessibility for audiences unfamiliar with te reo.

Aotearoa	New Zealand
Iwi	Tribe
Kaiāwhina	Contributors
Kaitiaki	One who leads and guides
Kaitiakitanga	Leading and guiding
Kanohi ki te kanohi	Face to face
Kaupapa Māori	Research for Māori, by Māori
Koha	A voluntary gift of thanks
Kotahitanga	Collectivity and unity
Māori	Indigenous people of Aotearoa/New Zealand
Manaakitanga	Hospitality, reciprocity and caring, role responsibility
Mana motuhake	Self-determination
Mātauranga Māori	Māori knowledge
Moko	Tattoo
Pākehā	New Zealander of European descent
Pūrākau	Story, narrative
Rangatiratanga	Self-determination, leadership
Tamariki	Children
Te ao Māori	The Māori world
Te reo	Language of the Indigenous people of Aotearoa
Tiakitanga	Unconditional love and commitment
Tikanga	Protocols, proper way of doing things, boundaries
Tīpuna	Ancestors (Eastern dialect)
Waiata	Songs, singing
Wairua	Spirit
Wairuatanga	Spirituality
Whakapapa	The scaffolding through which all things are connected is commonly used in the context of familial connectedness along genealogical lines.

(continued)

(continued)

Whānau	A social unit within Māori society typically consists of three–four generations of family. Pre-settler contact whānau lived in close proximity and undertook shared activities for the provision and prosperity of the collective group.
Whanaungatanga	System of practices rooted in mutual commitment that strengthens ties of kinship
Whanaungatanga hē	Practices or beliefs that are not in keeping with tikanga Māori. These tend to align more with coloniser ideology and have been inadvertently or purposefully misconceived over time as whanaungatanga.
Whanaungatanga iho	Practices that reflect the principles of whanaungatanga without manipulation and fulfil the promise of fostering well-being

References

Australian Institute of Health and Welfare. (2014). *Indigenous child safety*.

Barlow, C. (1991). *Tikanga Whakaaro: Key Concepts in Māori Culture*. Auckland: Oxford University Press.

Bishop, R. (1999). Kaupapa Maori research: An indigenous approach to creating knowledge. In N. Robertson (Ed.), *Maori and psychology: Research and practice—The proceedings of a symposium sponsored by the Maori and Psychology Research Unit*. Maori & Psychology Research Unit.

Draucker, C. B., & Martsolf, D. S. (2008). Storying childhood sexual abuse. *Qualitative Health Research, 18*(8), 1034–1048.

Du Mont, J., Kosa, D., Macdonald, S., Benoit, A., & Forte, T. (2017). A comparison of indigenous and non-indigenous survivors of sexual assault and their receipt of and satisfaction with specialised health care services. *PLoS ONE, 12*(11).

Durie, M. (2011). *Ngā Tini Whetū: Navigating Māori futures*. Huia Publishers.

Elizabeth, V. (2019). Personal communication.

Fanslow, J. L., Robinson, E. M., Crengle, S., & Perese, L. (2007). Prevalence of child sexual abuse reported by a cross-sectional sample of New Zealand women. *Child Abuse & Neglect, 31*.

Hamley, L., Groot, S., Grice, J. L., Gillon, A., Greaves, L., Manchi, M., & Clark, T. (2021). "You're the One That Was on Uncle's Wall!": Identity, Whanaungatanga and Connection for Takatāpui (LGBTQ+ Māori). *Genealogy, 5*(2).

HELP. (2022). *Sexual abuse statistics.* https://www.helpauckland.org.nz/sexual-abuse-statistics.html

Le Grice, J. (2019). Personal communication.

Le Grice, J., Braun, V., & Wetherell, M. (2017). "What I reckon is, is that like the love you give to your kids they'll give to someone else and so on and so on": Whanaungatanga and mātauranga Māori in practice. *New Zealand Journal of Psychology, 46*(3), 88–97.

Lee, J. (2009). Decolonising Māori narratives: Pūrākau as a method. *MAI Review,* (2), 12.

Lévi-Strauss, C. (1966). *The savage mind.* The University of Chicago Press.

McNatty, W., & Roa, T. (2002). Whanaungatanga: An illustration of the importance of cultural context. *He Puna Korero: Journal of Maori and Pacific Development, 3*(2), 88–96.

Metge J. (1995). *New Growth from Old: The Whānau in the Modern World.* Victoria University Press.

Mayhew, P., & Reilly, J. (2006). *The New Zealand crime and safety survey 2006.*

Mikaere, A. (1994). Maori women: Caught in the contradictions of a colonised reality. *Waikato Law Review, 6.*

Mikaere, A. (2011). *Colonising myths—Māori realities: he Rukuruku Whakaaro.* Huia Publishers.

Ministry of Justice. (2021). *Hāpaitia te Oranga Tangata.* https://www.justice.govt.nz/justice-sector-policy/key-initiatives/hapaitia-te-oranga-tangata/#:~:text=M%C4%81ori%20are%20overrepresented%20at%20every,of%20the%20New%20Zealand%20population

Ministry of Justice. (2022). *The New Zealand Crime and Victims Survey Key Findings Booklet: Cycle 4 November 2020 - November 2021.* https://www.justice.govt.nz/assets/20220628-NZCVS-Cycle-4-A5-Key-findings-booklet.pdf

Moewaka Barnes, H. (2000). Kaupapa Māori: Explaining the ordinary. *Pacific Health Dialogue, 7*(1), 13–16.

Moorfield, J. C. (2022a). *Te Aka: Māori dictionary, Hē.* https://maoridictionary.co.nz/search?idiom=&phrase=&proverb=&loan=&histLoanWords=&keywords=-he

Moorfield, J. C. (2022b). *Te Aka: Māori dictionary, Iho.* https://maoridictionary.co.nz/search?idiom=&phrase=&proverb=&loan=&histLoanWords=&keywords=iho

Morgan, D. H. (2011a). Locating 'Family Practices'. *Sociological Research Online, 16*(4), 14.

Morgan, D. H. (2011b). *Rethinking family practices.* Palgrave Macmillan.

Office of the Children's Commissioner. (2020). *Statistical snapshot: Pēpi Māori 0–3 months and the care and protection system.*

Pere, R. (1982). *Ako: Concepts and learning in the Māori tradition.* Te Kohanga Reo National Trust Board.

Pihama, L., & Lee-Morgan, J. (2022). *Tiakina te Pā Harakeke: Ancestral Knowledge and Tamariki Wellbeing* (L. Pihama & J. Lee-Morgan, Eds.). Huia Publishers.

Pihama, L., Nana, R. T., Cameron, N., Smith, C., Reid, J., & Southey, K. (2016). Māori cultural definitions of sexual violence. *Sexual Abuse in Australia and New Zealand, 7*(1), 43–51.

Rameka, L. (2016). Kia whakatōmuri te haere whakamua: 'I walk backwards into the future with my eyes fixed on my past'. *Contemporary Issues in Early Childhood, 17*(4), 387–398.

Ritchie, J. E. (1992). *Becoming bicultural.* Huia Publishers.

Sharman, T.-M. (2019). Personal communication.

Smart, C. (2007). *Personal life.* Polity Press.

Smith, G. (2012). Kaupapa Māori: The dangers of domestication. *New Zealand Journal of Educational Studies, 47*(2).

Smith, L. T. (2000). Kaupapa Māori research. In M. Battiste (Ed.), *Reclaiming indigenous voice and vision.* UBC Press.

Taonui, R. (2010). Mana Tamariki: Cultural alienation, Māori child homicide and abuse. *AlterNative: An International Journal of Indigenous Peoples, 6*(3), 187–202.

Tau, T. M. (2001). In defence of oral history: Whakapapa as a case study. *Karaka,* (17), 8–19.

Te Awekotuku, N. (2006). Mata Ora: Chiseling the living face—Dimensions of Maori Tattoo. In E. Edwards et al. (Eds.), *Sensible objects: Colonialism, museums and material culture.* Taylor & Francis Group.

Toi Iho. (2022). *About Toi Iho.* Retrieved July 24, 2022, from http://www.toi-iho.co.nz/about-toi-iho/

Tuhiwai Smith, L. (2012). *Decolonising methodologies: Research and indigenous peoples* (2nd ed.). Zed Books Ltd..

Walker, R. (2004). *Ka Whawhai Tonu Matou: Struggle without end* (Revised Ed.). Penguin Books.

Webb, R., & Shaw, R. M. (2011). Whanau, whakapapa and identity in experiences of organ donation and transplantation. *Sites: A Journal of Social Anthropology and Cultural Studies, 8*, 40–58.

Yancey, C. T., & Hansen, D. J. (2010). Relationship of personal, familial, and abuse-specific factors with outcome following childhood sexual abuse. *Aggression and Violent Behavior, 15*, 410–421.

5

Relational Contexts as Causal and Curative Pathways in Recurrent Suicidal Distress and Repeated Police Mental Health Act (Section 136) Detention

Claire Warrington

Introduction and Research Context

Relationships are a fundamental element of our human experience. Little wonder then, given the myriad complexities inherent to our lives, that the interplay between relationships and mental health is no less complex. This chapter examines how relationships over the life course impact beliefs and subsequently responses to experiences of interpersonal trauma that can lead to recurrent suicidality.

This chapter is based upon primary research that took place in South-East England between 2012–2018: Bendelow et al. (2019: Study One) and Warrington (2019a, b: Study Two). The studies were focussed on Section 136 Mental Health Act detention; an emergency police power

C. Warrington (✉)
University of York, York, UK
e-mail: claire.warrington@york.ac.uk

Z. Boden-Stuart, M. Larkin (eds.), *Relationships and Mental Health*,
https://doi.org/10.1007/978-3-031-50047-3_5

allowing the removal to a place of safety of a person who appears to be in immediate need of care or control owing to their mental state, to prevent that person causing imminent harm to themselves or others. Much research has demonstrated that most uses of this power relate to suicide prevention (e.g., Burgess et al., 2017; Laidlaw et al., 2010; Menkes & Bendelow, 2014). Furthermore, the police are recognised as having a role in responding to high-risk situations involving people experiencing suicidal crises in many countries (Clugston et al., 2023). However, it has only more recently begun to emerge that some people in England and Wales are repeatedly subject to Section 136 detention with high frequencies (Adewusi et al., 2022; Warrington, 2019a, b).

The research on which this chapter is based privileged the lived experience of crisis and detention, both studies were purposefully developed and conducted with a strong influence of co-production. In particular, Study Two incorporated a co-produced analysis with advisors who had themselves experienced crises arising from complex mental health problems helping to interpret the qualitative accounts of recurrent suicidal crises that had led to frequent police detentions.[1] Throughout the analyses, the pivotal role of relationships was continually highlighted by the advisors as the conduit through which experience had been mediated. Not only did the advisors indicate the theme of relationships as encompassing key points within the data but also, when speaking of their own lived experiences of crises and help-seeking, here too were a multitude of ways in which relationships had influenced incidents, care, and outcomes. The research demonstrated that for some women who had initially survived interpersonal traumas, recurrent suicidality was rooted in relational complexities arising from these traumas not being addressed. The data further showed that relationships also held the potential to provide a reparative means to break the dangerous cycles of repeated suicide attempts into which these women had become enmeshed.

This chapter presents the model of recurrent suicidality which was developed in Study Two. A case study derived from a composite of the

[1] On completion of data collection, consultation workshops reviewing anonymised excerpts of the interview data were held with members of a research advisory forum for people who identified as having lived experience relevant to the Personality, Emergency mental health Care and Complexity (PECC) research theme of Sussex Partnership NHS Foundation Trust.

accounts shared by research participants in both studies illustrates how the model operates and indicates critical moments that could be seen as turning points. 'Lou' does not exist, but her story is real.

A Note on Terminology

Suicidality

This chapter uses the terms suicidal distress and suicidality to encompass suicidal thoughts and actions as well as deliberate self-harm. The use of this shorthand has been adopted primarily for brevity, but also because little distinction is commonly made by police officers in deciding whether to detain an individual, or the lay public who often alert the police to the situation. It should however be noted that there are significant differences in types of self-harm; a deliberate act of producing physical injury, which may not have the intent of ending life. Indeed, self-harm can at times be a demonstration of an individual's desire to remain alive; experiencing physical pain to ground themselves from psychological pain and remain connected to life (see for example Chandler, 2013; Chaney, 2017; Simopoulou & Chandler, 2020).

In the cases of those who came into frequent contact with emergency services through repeated suicide attempts, participants spoke candidly about differences in the aims of their actions on different occasions. Whilst self-harming was a common occurrence within periods of distress that drove multiple self-destructive and risky behaviours, for these individuals it was sometimes part of attempts to end life but at others more of an attempt to cope and remain alive.

Likewise, suicidal thoughts and actions can be seen as occurring on a spectrum that can differ both between and within individual experience (Joiner, 2005). Although suicidal thoughts may not always be acted upon, prior suicide attempts are one of the greatest risk factors for a future suicide completion and self-harm can likewise be a predictor of future fatal suicide (Skegg, 2005).

Personality Disorder Diagnoses

Many of the study participants who had been repeatedly detained had either been diagnosed with borderline or emotionally unstable personality disorder or were treated as though assumed to have such a diagnosis. These terms were also commonly used by non-medical professionals, including police. Several participants from both studies had over time received conflicting diagnoses and some had been assessed by personality disorder specialists as not having a personality disorder at all. These highly vexed diagnoses are discussed subsequently herein and a greater consideration of some of the difficulties attached to these diagnoses are provided in the original publications. The terms borderline or emotionally unstable personality disorder are used in this chapter as they were presented in the original contexts and the contraction B/EUPD is adopted to cover both formal diagnoses and the 'unofficial' assumption that an individual who has been repeatedly detained would have such a diagnosis. The case study presented demonstrates how B/EUPD is "a disorder of relationship, not of personality" (Lester, 2013, p. 74) as it arises where adaptive skills developed to negotiate and survive detrimental relational contexts become fixed and problematic in later life.

A Relational Model of Recurrent Suicidality

Study Two developed the relational model of recurrent suicidality (see Fig. 5.1) drawing on Realist Evaluation (Pawson & Tilley, 1997). This approach seeks to understand a situation by articulating Contexts, generative Mechanisms (the elements that are activated in that context) and the resultant Outcomes, which are triggered by that interaction. The model is presented using Dalkin et al.'s (2015) conceptualisation to disaggregate 'Mechanism' into its dyadic constituent components of Resource and Reasoning. Realist evaluation considers that outcomes are caused by participants' reasoning (responses) to something that is introduced to a field of study (resource) rather than the resource itself. Thus, in the context of recurrent suicidality and repeated detention, the

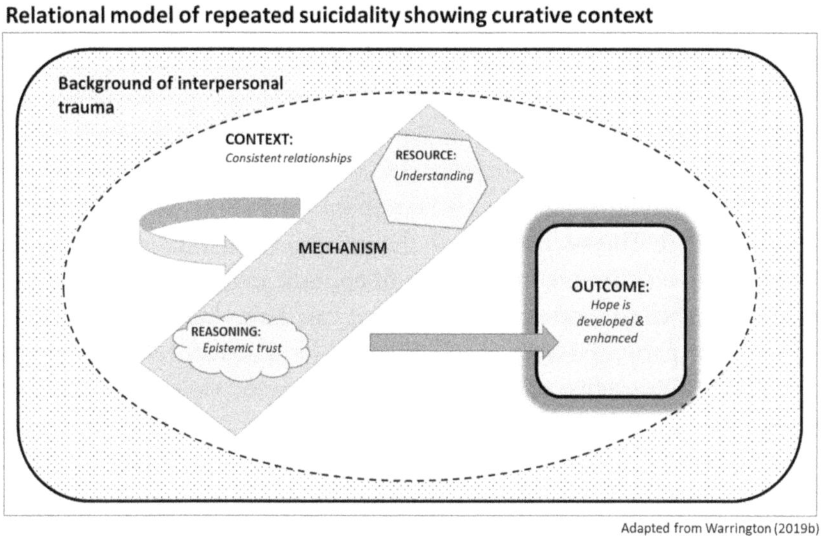

Fig. 5.1 A relational model of repeated suicidality showing the curative context

reasoning was identified as epistemic trust,[2] which was coupled with the resource of understanding as its dyadic pairing. This mechanism operated within the context of relationships to influence suicidality by either enhancing or impeding the outcome, which was identified as hope.

Accordingly, the mechanism was conceived as having a two-way operation, such that in the genesis of recurrent suicidality, detrimental contexts (i.e., poor, inconsistent, or harmful relationships) fractured the individuals' concept (understanding) of themselves and others and their capacity to trust. Conversely, in what were labelled curative contexts (illustrated in Fig. 5.1) positive relationships provided an environment in which an individual received understanding that enabled them to develop epistemic trust, and to therefore break away from self-destructive cycles as hope was triggered or enhanced.

[2] Epistemic trust is the capacity of an individual to believe new social information can be relevant and reliable enough to integrate into their belief system (Fonagy & Allison, 2014). It has been theorised as underpinning 'borderline pathology' (Fonagy et al., 2015).

Relationships: The Critical Scaffold to Psychosocial Development

Early relational interactions with significant people in our lives heavily influence a range of later outcomes by shaping patterns of thought and behaviour which form guiding beliefs about others, the world, and ourselves within it. This occurs on both the micro-level of individual encounters and through an ongoing process of episodic evaluation. In this way, events from childhood and adolescence can have long-lasting consequences. In particular, Adverse Childhood Experiences (ACEs) are ten serious negative events, such as exposure to domestic violence, emotional neglect and household dysfunction, that can have a cumulative impact and are associated with poor physical and mental health in adulthood (Dube et al., 2001; Felitti et al., 1998). The following case study illustrates how these factors can operate.

Lou is 36 years old. She describes her childhood as "not a terribly happy one." Her father was an inconsistent presence through her early years, and she later discovered his multiple affairs were the reason for his frequent absences from the family home. Her mother drank heavily, and as an only child Lou often bore the brunt of her verbally aggressive and occasionally violent outbursts. Whenever Lou became visibly distressed at this abuse, her mother would condemn her for being histrionic. As a result of these circumstances, Lou learned to be an appeaser, to rapidly gauge the atmosphere in the home and how intoxicated her mother was. When her father was present, she would be on continued alert to mannerisms and tones of voice that indicated friction between her parents and warning signs that another row was imminent. Lou was an intelligent child and performed well at school despite her attendance being patchy "whenever things were bad at home." Reflecting back, Lou acknowledges her early perfectionism likely distracted her teachers from more closely examining her absences from school and home circumstances. Lou recalls that she did have intermittent contact with social workers through her childhood, but she had rapidly learned how to give "the right" answers to ensure she didn't provoke any more problems through involvement from outsiders that her parents considered intrusive.

When Lou was 14, her mother began an affair with a neighbour who would come to the house whenever her father was away. Within a short period of time his interest in Lou became apparent so she began to seek ways to avoid going home. Lou began hanging out and drinking with older peers. Mostly, she sought a sense of acceptance, trying to fit in with a group to which she didn't really feel she belonged. She was flattered when one of the popular boys in the group appeared to take an interest in her and she automatically sought to avoid rejection through compliance. Lou fell pregnant shortly before she turned 15. She confirmed her suspicions with a stolen pregnancy test a few weeks after her birthday. Despite being terrified of what would happen when people found out, as the pregnancy progressed, Lou says she began to nurture some thoughts of having someone on whom she could lavish the affection she herself craved.

Her mother's boyfriend continued to make sexualised comments and advances without her mother appearing to notice. As a result, Lou increasingly stayed overnight with various school friends until one girl's parents picked up that something was wrong and, although she wouldn't expand on why, she accepted their offer that she stay with them "for a while." Despite being glad of the refuge, Lou worried that the family may change their minds at any stage, especially if her pregnancy was discovered and so whilst feeling physically safe at last, she remained vigilant for signs that this security would be rescinded. When Lou lost her baby, she says she was too scared to seek help even if she had known where to turn, so she started truanting and drinking again to dull the feelings of guilt and sorrow.

Lou experienced multiple ACEs and the relationships with her parents would have impacted her attachment style (Ainsworth, 1964). Whereas secure attachments are likely to be fostered through consistent and appropriate carer responses and provide good foundations for emotional and social development; abusive or inconsistent behaviour from a child's carers, such as Lou experienced from both her parents, can lead to insecure (anxious or avoidant) attachment with a resultant belief system that holds others as untrustworthy (Ainsworth et al., 1978). Belief systems engendered by attachment can continue to influence relationships throughout the life course and impact a range of health and social factors, including increasing likelihood of problematic substance misuse and contact with the criminal justice system (Green et al., 2020). In Lou's case, these elements manifested in her relationships with her peers and other adults around her, as well as her burgeoning issues with alcohol. Despite accessing a positive environment when she moved in with her friend, her prior experiences had already taught her that adults were unreliable and that feeling safe was likely only a temporary state. This epistemic mistrust (a lack of capacity to consider new social knowledge: Fonagy & Allison, 2014) meant that Lou was not able to learn to feel secure with her friend's parents and so kept them at a distance, and crucially felt unable to confide in anyone about her pregnancy.

Unable to gain Lou's trust enough for her to open up to them, eventually her friend's parents arranged for her to go to stay with relatives in another part of the country. She was enrolled in a local college, and it was agreed by all involved that a fresh start would be good for her. Lou settled into her new home and although by her account she didn't form what she would call any close bonds with either her contemporaries or her relatives, her attendance at college was much improved and she engaged well enough with her studies to gain a place on a nursing degree. But at university Lou found herself once more in a cohort of heavy drinkers amongst whom her own excessive alcohol use was normalised.

During her degree, Lou began seeing an older man who worked on the campus security team. The two were married shortly after she graduated, and their first child was born a little while later. Her husband joined the police and his mother, who was recently retired, helped with childcare when Lou returned to work. For a few years she recalls that her life seemed settled and although her husband became increasingly controlling around their household finances and Lou socialising with colleagues, she continued to perform well at work and was well-respected. Lou derived a great deal of satisfaction from her job and her career progressed well. However, at home she felt she was not a good enough parent, and she experienced a constant anxiety over her son, which kept her on-edge much of the time.

Lou's marriage gradually deteriorated during this time. She would later recognise her husband's criticisms of her parenting as part of his controlling abusive behaviour, which served to undermine her confidence, but his mother was supportive of her and the two had developed a closeness. Lou's drinking was "under control" in the first few years of her son's life, and she felt that focussing on him and work was enough. Approaching the tenth anniversary of her miscarriage, Lou found out she was expecting again. As she had been with her son, she was gripped with fear that she would lose another child. Finally, one evening while her husband was working a night shift, she confided in her mother-in-law about what had happened with her teenage pregnancy; it was the first time Lou had spoken about her lost baby. Returning to her home later that night, her mother-in-law was knocked down and killed by a drunk driver.

Another way in which ACEs are likely to impact adult life is through emotional dysregulation in adolescence and later life, the results of which can be seen through peer and adult relationships, disengagement from education, and reckless behaviour including substance misuse and sexual risk-taking (Sousa et al., 2011). These factors mediated through insecure attachments can impact subsequent relationships. Experiencing domestic abuse can also give rise to complexities in attachments (Bartholomew & Allison, 2006; Bartholomew et al., 2001). Furthermore, there is a broadly recognised intergenerational effect of childhood exposure to abuse (Livings et al., 2022). It is likely these experiences all impact the individual's belief system. Lou described growing up with a degree of hypervigilance, being alert for indicators of rejection, and this may also have made her more vulnerable to the impact of moral injury (Shay, 2014). This has been hypothesised to be a core component in developing a traumatic response through the betrayal of trust in certain 'high stakes' situations.

Moral injury and the resulting post-traumatic response can have long-lasting, detrimental consequences on future psychological states when not addressed, driving down hope by fundamentally altering the individual's worldview. The failure of Lou's parents to protect her as a child and her husband's abuse represented fundamental violations of trust. These detrimental relational contexts shaped Lou's beliefs and understanding of herself and others, which was seen in study participants who expressed self-blame for their suicidality. This was coupled with epistemic mistrust, which in the model is represented by the belief that there was no source of help or support that could offer the foundation for a meaningful recovery from despair. In turn this culminated in a sense of futility, labelled as hopelessness.

Lou describes the period following her mother in-law's death as the first time in which she "totally lost it." She is unclear about events during the rest of her pregnancy but remembers being entirely overwhelmed by fierce emotions that included feeling responsible for the deaths of her mother-in-law and first child. Lou was admitted to hospital following an overdose shortly after her daughter was born. Over the next few years, Lou continued to drink heavily, she developed an eating disorder and her self-harming escalated as she began to cut and burn herself. She lost her job and her husband had become physically as well as verbally abusive; he continually called her an unfit mother. When they separated, he took the children and Lou became increasingly suicidal, believing herself to be a failed parent and that her children would be better off without her.

Lou's first police Mental Health Act detention happened when a shop worker refused to sell her alcohol as she was already intoxicated. She responded aggressively and left the shop knocking over a counter display. Officers found her walking towards a motorway and she later heard they had received a call from a cyclist who had been concerned about her. When the police arrived Lou recalls thinking her husband had sent them and trying to run away in terror. The officers believed Lou to be a risk to herself and detained her under Section 136 of the Mental Health Act. Lou was admitted to a psychiatric hospital. Subsequently, during ward rounds, the psychiatrist stated she could be discharged as they had made a diagnosis. When asked by a colleague what the diagnosis was, he replied, "Emotionally Unstable Personality Disorder."

After receiving a diagnosis, Lou hoped at first that she may begin to receive support but instead found that professionals now seemed colder towards her. Her suicidality meant she had begun to be detained repeatedly under Section 136 and her initial reaction of terror at the sight of police approaching her persisted so that she often tried to flee or fight restraint when she was being detained. During these years she was frequently taken to the Accident & Emergency Department but rarely encountered sympathetic healthcare staff. Instead, she was often treated with bluntness that she noticed worsened if her professional background became known. She overheard multiple conversations about her during these years, learning she had been labelled as a "runner." On another occasion someone in an Accident & Emergency Department said that as a former nurse, Lou of all people should understand the pressures they were under and ought to know better than to waste time with attention seeking. Lou wanted to explain that she wasn't trying to waste anyone's time and didn't want to keep being detained as was often implied, but that she genuinely wanted to die, believing she had nothing to live for.

Distress as a Relational Disorder

Sadly, Lou's experiences are far from atypical as the stigma and discriminatory practices that Sulzer (2015) has adroitly labelled '*de facto demedicalisation*' are widespread. Psychiatrists have admitted a reticence to inform patients that they have made a diagnosis of B/EUPD (Sisti et al., 2016) and personality disorder remains broadly a "Diagnosis of Exclusion" (NHS, 2003). Such examples are among the reasons these diagnoses remain highly problematic, as do the uncertainties surrounding the validity of personality disorder as a construct (Bendelow, 2010).

Participants in both studies spoke of having received conflicting diagnoses, with specialists having assessed some as not having a personality disorder at all. Many described being treated as though they had this diagnosis apparently solely based on their recurrent suicidality. Study Two found that people with recorded diagnoses of personality disorder accounted for over half all repeated detentions, whilst the narrative accounts revealed the significant impact of interpersonal trauma and illustrated another longstanding criticism of B/EUPD. The incidence of traumatic backgrounds amongst those diagnosed with B/EUPD has been reported to be as much as 90% (Yen et al., 2002) which gives rise to the critique that these diagnoses serve primarily to pathologise survivors of abuse; effectively attributing culpability for the psychological consequences of trauma to victims (Shaw & Proctor, 2005). Moreover, this misattribution is often internalised, as reflected in Lou's feelings of guilt tied to the bereavements she experienced. Self-blame was a key component of interviewees' accounts, as were mentions of these views having been reinforced through negative interactions with professionals. Disregarding the authenticity of distress or dismissing it as attention-seeking or manipulation signals that the individual is unworthy or unable to be helped (Lester, 2013).

Mental health workers interviewed in Study One talked about people who were repeatedly detained and diagnosed with B/EUPD as not being "really ill" (Bendelow et al., 2019, p. 98). Indeed, people who have self-harmed or attempted suicide commonly encounter negative responses from staff in physical healthcare settings, particularly emergency departments (Warm et al., 2002) and participants in both studies also reported this. Far from being a new phenomenon, Jeffery (1979, p. 92) observed doctors referring to patients who had attempted suicide as being part of "the usual rubbish," which also included patients who were intoxicated. Here too, questions around the validity and potential harm of B/EUPD arise, as both suicidality and problematic substance use are recognised consequences of the harms of ACEs and unresolved adult trauma, as well being considered potential indicators of B/EUPD (American Psychiatric Association, 2013).

There are likely to be reasons for the negative responses in healthcare settings beyond simply condemnation of the individual, including lack of understanding, discomfort and uncertainty around roles and boundaries between care and control, and fear of worsening situations that are not likely to be resolved as quickly as some physical health problems (McHale & Felton, 2010). Whatever the reasons underlying apparent unsympathetic responses, research participants in Study One were clear that the effect is often a significant deterioration of trust in healthcare professionals and a reluctance to seek help in future incidents. Whether in times of distress, following self-harm or suicide attempts, or more generally during planned interactions such as appointments with mental health workers, the responses individuals received from professionals had a critical role in the relational context model. Furthermore, multiple other studies have highlighted the importance of relational factors in such encounters (Goodall et al., 2019; Haigh, 2005; Jones & Mason, 2002).

Conclusion: The Reparational Potential of Relationships

Lou's story describes the impact of detrimental relational contexts in both her childhood and later life instilling and reinforcing negative beliefs about herself and others and rendering her vulnerable to recurrent suicidality. Negative encounters, especially with healthcare staff were experienced as retraumatising and further diminished her ability to build constructive, trusting relationships that could support her to break the dangerous cycle of suicidal crises. Conversely, the model illustrated at the start of this chapter shows how curative relational contexts that provide consistent, supportive relationships offering understanding and facilitating the development of epistemic trust were fundamental to the trajectory away from recurrent suicidality. The research showed how a diagnosis of B/EUPD could be positive where it facilitated access to such an environment.

The most obvious difference between participants for whom recurrent suicidality and repeated detentions were past experiences and those who were still caught in cycles of despair was engagement with a service that was built on relational principles, centred around attachment theory, and tailored to support people with a diagnosis of personality disorder (although predominantly the term 'emotional intensity' was used; Warrington, 2019a). Over time, within this context of consistent and secure, positive relationships, participants were able to engage with the understanding offered by staff at the service. This was demonstrated both in psychoeducational work examining how prior experiences had impacted beliefs and led to self-destructive patterns of thought and behaviour, as well as being embodied in the practice of all staff. As one participant explained, this meant she could ring into the service when in crisis and the receptionist would know in a few words to put her through to a keyworker who could help her de-escalate without protracted explanations. In contrast, participants reported numerous examples of the reverse when trying to access support from mainstream mental health teams. A key finding from the first study was that those who were detained repeatedly were typically known to mental health services but were considered to have disengaged from these services (e.g., not responding to attempts to make contact or were no longer attending appointments) many participants cited poor relationships with care coordinators as a significant reason for this.

The whole service understanding was a critical factor of the curative relational context. Positive relationships and social support outside the home can serve as a key protective factor against the negative consequences of childhood trauma (Cheong et al., 2017), specifically the presence of an 'always available adult' who is consistent and trusted, has the capacity to ameliorate the associated harms of ACEs (Bellis et al., 2017).

It was notable that each of the participants who were not receiving adequate support described one or two lasting good relationships, but that these were not sufficient to protect from the recurrent suicidal crises which led to their repeated detentions. For example, one participant in this group spoke of a therapist who really understood her but said that seeing him once a week didn't alter her overall circumstances. Another participant spoke about a community mental health team care co-ordinator, whom she couldn't praise highly enough, but said she had still found living unbearable prior to joining the support service. It is therefore hypothesised that once trauma had been embedded in adulthood, individual positive supportive relationships could not fulfil their full reparative potential, but rather that an "always available community" (Warrington, 2019a, p. 215) was needed, such as that provided by the support service described in the study.

Within such a curative relational context, epistemic trust was fostered from understanding, which enabled the restructuring of harmful beliefs, and ultimately the development of a sense of hope, which was evidenced through participants' future focussed comments. Naturally, hope, or its absence, has a crucial role in suicide, which has been well articulated in numerous studies and models (Benson et al., 2016; Joiner, 2005; Williams, 2001). Levi-Belz et al. (2013) suggested the psychological vulnerabilities inherent to those with insecure attachments increase an individual's experience of mental pain, that in combination with triggers such as depression, can exacerbate hopelessness and suicidal ideation.

The relational model discussed herein contributes an understanding of how these elements can operate within the overarching context of unresolved interpersonal trauma, to trigger recurrent suicidality from detrimental contexts or to offer a route to recovery when a community-level consistent curative relational context can be accessed.

References

Adewusi, L., Mark, I., Wells, P., & O'Brien, A. (2022). A retrospective cohort study describing characteristics of those repeatedly detained under Section 136 of the Mental Health Act over a 5-year period and the association with past abuse. *Medicine, Science and the Law, 62*(2), 124–133.

Ainsworth, M. (1964). The Bowlby-Ainsworth attachment theory. *Behavioral and Brain Sciences, 1*(3), 436–438.

Ainsworth, M. D. S., Blehar, M. C., Waters, E., & Wall, S. (1978). *Patterns of attachment*. Lawrence Erlbaum Associates, Inc.

American Psychiatric Association. (2013). *Diagnostic and statistical manual of mental disorders* (5th ed.). American Psychiatric Association.

Bartholomew, K., & Allison, C. J. (2006). An attachment perspective on abusive dynamics in intimate relationships. In M. Mikulincer & G. S. Goodman (Eds.), *Dynamics of romantic love: Attachment, caregiving, and sex* (pp. 102–127). Guilford Press.

Bartholomew, K., Henderson, A., & Dutton, D. (2001). Insecure attachment and abusive intimate relationships. In C. Clulow (Ed.), *Adult attachment and couple psychotherapy: The 'secure base' in practice and research* (pp. 43–61). Brunner-Routledge.

Bellis, M. A., Hardcastle, K., Ford, K., Hughes, K., Ashton, K., Quigg, Z., & Butler, N. (2017). Does continuous trusted adult support in childhood impart life-course resilience against adverse childhood experiences-a retrospective study on adult health-harming behaviours and mental well-being. *BMC Psychiatry, 17*(1), 1–12.

Bendelow, G. (2010). Ethical aspects of personality disorders. *Current Opinion in Psychiatry, 23*(6), 546–549.

Bendelow, G., Warrington, C. A., Jones, A. M., & Markham, S. (2019). Police detentions of 'mentally disordered persons': A multi-method investigation of section 136 use in Sussex. *Medicine, Science and the Law, 59*(2), 95–103.

Benson, O., Gibson, S., Boden, Z. V., & Owen, G. (2016). Exhausted without trust and inherent worth: A model of the suicide process based on experiential accounts. *Social Science & Medicine, 163*, 126–134. https://doi.org/10.1016/j.socscimed.2016.06.045

Burgess, J. L., White, S. J., & O'Brien, A. (2017). Retrospective cohort follow-up study of individuals detained under Section 136. *BJPsych Open, 3*(6), 281–284.

Chandler, A. (2013). Inviting pain? Pain, dualism and embodiment in narratives of self-injury. *Sociology of Health & Illness, 35*(5), 716–730. https://doi.org/10.1111/j.1467-9566.2012.01523.x

Chaney, S. (2017). *Psyche on the skin: A history of self-harm*. Reaktion Books.

Cheong, E., Sinnott, C., Dahly, D., & Kearney, P. (2017). Adverse childhood experiences (ACEs) and later-life depression: Perceived social support as a potential protective factor. *BMJ Open, 7*, e013228.

Clugston, B., Meurk, C., Harris, M., Burgess, P., & Heffernan, E. (2023). Persons with mental disorders and suicidality in crisis or high-risk situations involving police negotiation: A systematic review. *Psychiatry, Psychology and Law*, 1–19.

Dalkin, S. M., Greenhalgh, J., Jones, D., Cunningham, B., & Lhussier, M. (2015). What's in a mechanism? Development of a key concept in realist evaluation. *Implementation Science, 10*(1), 1–7.

Dube, S. R., Anda, R. F., Felitti, V. J., Chapman, D. P., Williamson, D. F., & Giles, W. H. (2001). Childhood abuse, household dysfunction, and the risk of attempted suicide throughout the life span: Findings from the Adverse Childhood Experiences study. *Journal of the American Medical Association, 286*(24), 3089–3096. https://doi.org/10.1001/JAMA.286.24.3089

Felitti, V. J., Anda, R. F., Nordenberg, D., Williamson, D. F., Spitz, A. M., Edwards, V., & Marks, J. S. (1998). Relationship of childhood abuse and household dysfunction to many of the leading causes of death in adults: The Adverse Childhood Experiences (ACE) Study. *American Journal of Preventive Medicine, 14*(4), 245–258.

Fonagy, P., & Allison, E. (2014). The role of mentalizing and epistemic trust in the therapeutic relationship. *Psychotherapy, 51*(3), 372.

Fonagy, P., Luyten, P., & Allison, E. (2015). Epistemic petrification and the restoration of epistemic trust: A new conceptualization of borderline personality disorder and its psychosocial treatment. *Journal of Personality Disorders, 29*(5), 575–609.

Goodall, T., Newton, E., & Larkin, M. (2019). What are the critical incidents that affect how people cope with being detained under Section 136 of the Mental Health Act (1983, 2007)? *International Journal of Psychiatry in Clinical Practice, 23*(3), 194–206.

Green, J., Berry, K., Danquah, A., & Pratt, D. (2020). The role of psychological and social factors in the relationship between attachment and suicide: A systematic review. *Clinical Psychology & Psychotherapy, 27*(4), 463–488.

Haigh, R. (2005) The Trouble with Modernisation: *We Need Better Relationships Not Policies and Procedures Mental Health Review Journal 10*(3) 3–7 https://doi.org/10.1108/13619322200500022

Jeffery, R. (1979). Normal rubbish: Deviant patients in casualty departments. *Sociology of Health & Illness, 1*(1), 90–107.

Joiner, T. E. (2005). *Why people die by suicide*. Harvard University Press.

Jones, S. L., & Mason, T. (2002). Quality of treatment following police detention of mentally disordered offenders. *Journal of Psychiatric and Mental Health Nursing, 9*(1), 73–80.

Laidlaw, J., Pugh, D., Riley, G., & Hovey, N. (2010). The use of Section 136 (Mental Health Act 1983) in Gloucestershire. *Medicine, Science and the Law, 50*(1), 29–33.

Lester, R. J. (2013). Lessons from the borderline: Anthropology, psychiatry, and the risks of being human. *Feminism & Psychology, 23*(1), 70–77.

Levi-Belz, Y., Gvion, Y., Horesh, N., & Apter, A. (2013). Attachment patterns in medically serious suicide attempts: The mediating role of self-disclosure and loneliness. *Suicide and Life-threatening Behavior, 43*(5), 511–522.

Livings, M. S., Hsiao, V., & Withers, M. (2022). Breaking the cycle of family violence: A critique of family violence interventions. *Trauma, Violence, & Abuse*, 15248380221098049.

McHale, J., & Felton, A. (2010). Self-harm: What's the problem? A literature review of the factors affecting attitudes towards self-harm. *Journal of Psychiatric and Mental Health Nursing, 17*(8), 732–740.

Menkes, D. B., & Bendelow, G. A. (2014). Diagnosing vulnerability and "dangerousness": Police use of section 136 in England and Wales. *Journal of Public Mental Health, 13*(2), 70–82. https://doi.org/10.1108/JPMH-09-2012-0001

NHS National Institute for Mental Health in England. (2003). *Personality disorder: No longer a diagnosis of exclusion*. NIMH(E).

Pawson, R., & Tilley, N. (1997). *Realistic evaluation*. Sage.

Shaw, C., & Proctor, G. (2005). Women at the margins: A critique of the diagnosis of borderline personality disorder. *Feminism & Psychology, 15*(4), 483–490.

Shay, J. (2014). Moral injury. *Psychoanalytic Psychology, 31*(2), 182.

Simopoulou, Z., & Chandler, A. (2020). Self-harm as an attempt at self-care. *European Journal for Qualitative Research in Psychotherapy, 10*, 110–120.

Sisti, D., Segal, A. G., Siegel, A. M., Johnson, R., & Gunderson, J. (2016). Diagnosing, disclosing, and documenting borderline personality disorder: A survey of psychiatrists' practices. *Journal of Personality Disorders, 30*(6), 848–856.

Skegg, K. (2005). Self-harm. *The Lancet, 366*(9495), 1471–1483.

Sousa, C., Herrenkohl, T. I., Moylan, C. A., Tajima, E. A., Klika, J. B., Herrenkohl, R. C., & Russo, M. J. (2011). Longitudinal study on the effects of child abuse and children's exposure to domestic violence, parent-child attachments, and antisocial behavior in adolescence. *Journal of Interpersonal Violence, 26*(1), 111–136.

Sulzer, S. H. (2015). Does "difficult patient" status contribute to de facto demedicalization? The case of borderline personality disorder. *Social Science & Medicine, 142*, 82–89.

Warm, A., Murray, C., & Fox, J. (2002). Who helps? Supporting people who self-harm. *Journal of Mental Health, 11*(2), 121–130.

Warrington, C. (2019a). *Frequent detainees under Section 136 of the Mental Health Act (1983): Lived experience and service perspectives on repeated detention*. Doctoral thesis, University of Brighton.

Warrington, C. (2019b). Repeated police Mental Health Act detentions in England and Wales: Trauma and recurrent suicidality. *International Journal of Environmental Research and Public Health, 16*(23), 4786.

Williams, J. M. G. (2001). *The cry of pain*. Penguin.

Yen, S., Shea, M. T., Battle, C. L., Johnson, D. M., Zlotnick, C., Dolan-Sewell, R., ... & McGLASHAN, T. H. (2002). Traumatic exposure and posttraumatic stress disorder in borderline, schizotypal, avoidant, and obsessive-compulsive personality disorders: fingings from the collaborative longitudinal personality disorders study. *The Journal of nervous and mental disease, 190*(8), 510–518.

6

Working Through Relational Trauma: An Exploration of Narratives of Lived Experiences of Trauma and Recovery

Penn Smith and Divine Charura

As professionals we share many years of experience working with individuals who present with complex trauma. This informs our understanding and application of theory, research, and counselling practice. In this work we share a particular focus on understanding the meaning that individuals give to their experiences, and on working with trauma through relational means. Through our professional roles we have noted the devastating effects of trauma and the impact this can have on an individual's capacity to relate to self and others. However, we have also witnessed the importance of reparative relationships in the pursuit of easing psychological distress.

Many agree that the quality of the therapeutic relationship is an important factor for success when working with individuals experiencing *Relational Trauma* (Charura & Smith, 2023; Cooper, 2007; Finlay, 2016; Paul & Charura, 2014). Thus, our main focus is on relationships and experiences which offer the right conditions for transformation to enable

P. Smith (✉) • D. Charura
York St John University, York, UK
e-mail: p.smith2@yorksj.ac.uk

Z. Boden-Stuart, M. Larkin (eds.), *Relationships and Mental Health*,
https://doi.org/10.1007/978-3-031-50047-3_6

growth and change in one's felt sense of self and being-in-the-world. This chapter is informed by relational-centred, existential-phenomenological theoretical perspectives which assert that all humans have a built-in propensity to grow to their full potential when specific conditions are met. However, personal problems and trauma arise in and through relationality thereby interrupting connection with self and others. To start with we offer some definitions below of *relational trauma* and consider how issues can arise in and through relationality.

Understanding Psychological Trauma in Adulthood

We will firstly explore the current definitions of trauma and consider some contemporary background literature. The American Psychological Association (APA) defines trauma as "an emotional response to a terrible event like an accident, rape, or natural disaster" (APA, 2022). Trauma by its very definition is deeply distressing and disturbing, and leaves traces on our emotions, thoughts, and physiology, as well as impacting our capacity for intimacy and well-being (van der Kolk, 2014).

Over the last three decades, a growing body of literature has contributed to our understanding of trauma (Farina et al., 2019). In general, trauma literature has highlighted conceptualisations of psychotraumatology across the lifespan and made links between developmental trauma and the long-term psychological consequences of cumulative traumatic childhood experiences (Farina et al., 2019; van der Kolk, 1996). Furthermore, there has been critique of the international diagnostic systems for their failure to account for diverse clinical presentations of trauma which manifest in adulthood (Cloitre et al., 2011; Farina et al., 2019; van der Kolk, 1996). In this chapter, we wish to use 'trauma' in the broader sense that underpins these critiques. This use of 'trauma' is a meaningful and psychologically-coherent concept for us because it captures the diverse pathways that can connect a psychologically threatening experience to a subsequent difficulty with psychological wellbeing. Specifically, we propose and use the term *relational trauma* to include the experience of the severing, fragmenting, and/or violating of a significant relationship(s).

Our broader use of the trauma concept, and within that, our more specific focus on relational trauma, are based upon research that highlights the links between developmental trauma and its role in the aetiology of numerous mental disorders. Some of this prior research has focused on *cumulative developmental trauma (CDT)*, which is also referred to as *early relational trauma* (Isobel et al., 2017). In their conceptual analysis of psychological trauma in the context of familial relationships, Isobel et al. (2017) highlighted how the interpersonal nature of traumatic experiences (cumulative stressful and traumatic events that occur repeatedly over a period of time) can be the root of trauma. In line with this, others have noted the familial relational aspect of trauma and how psychological distress and some psychological disorders can be the result of traumatisation in early years of life. This has been conceptualised as *attachment trauma* (Isobel et al., 2017; Farina et al., 2019). Literature which expands on this includes, for example, the recognition of how *cumulative developmental/attachment trauma* contributes to dissociative disorders, personality disorders, and post-traumatic stress disorder (PTSD) (Farina et al., 2019; Sar, 2011; Terock et al., 2016; Williamson et al., 2017). As a consequence, there are good grounds for arguing that experiences and relationships in early life can have important consequences for psychological wellbeing in adulthood.

We have arrived at our understanding of relational trauma, which extends beyond this core argument, through Interpretative Phenomenological Analysis (IPA) as described in the next section.

Methodological Approach

This chapter draws from two research studies. One was conducted with 15 service users[1] from a United Kingdom (UK) mental health rehabilitation and recovery service (Smith et al., 2021), and one with 12

[1] Within the UK the term Service User typically describes any individual who has accessed or is eligible to access health and social care services. In other contexts, the words clients, patients etc. may be used.

asylum-seekers and refugees based in the UK (Taylor et al., 2020). Creative methodologies were used to capture the uniqueness and depth of lived experiences of the participants. Interview transcripts were analysed using interpretative phenomenological analysis (IPA). IPA has previously proved successful as a method for analysing semi-structured interviews along with creative data collection methods (Lachal et al., 2012) and was used to analyse the interview transcripts.

IPA, a popular health psychology research method, moves away from observational research towards a more constructed understanding that gives voice to individual experience (Brocki & Wearden, 2006). Grounded within phenomenology and hermeneutics, IPA aims to understand individual's experiences and how sense making occurs (Shaw, 2010; Smith et al., 2009, 2022). In engaging with the hermeneutic cycle, researchers adopt a reflexive attitude, one where self and other are examined within the research process. This reflects the relational-centred, existential-phenomenological approach we are adopting. Relatively small sample sizes are the norm in IPA (Smith et al., 2009, 2022). Furthermore, the strength of IPA lies in its ability to provide in-depth idiographic insights that are unique to each individual participant, and whilst also enabling conceptualisation of shared themes common across the range of lived experiences (Smith & Osborn, 2008).

Case Studies

Our work draws on relational-centred and existential-phenomenological concepts that have been written about in depth elsewhere (see Finlay, 2016; Paul & Charura, 2014; Spinelli, 1997/2006, 2015; van Deurzen, 2012; Yalom, 1980, 1989/2012). We might characterise these concepts most concisely by saying that they are primarily concerned with equipping researchers and therapists with the tools to understand aspects of the world *as it is lived* from the perspective of *those who are living it*. Working in this way, we are presenting a condensed summary of different case studies focusing on trauma and psychological distress/dis-ease in different contexts. The people we are referring to as 'participants' are mental health service users (Case Study 6.1) and asylum-seekers and refugees (Case Study 6.2).

Case Study 6.1

The study (Smith et al., 2021) was based in a United Kingdom (UK) service that is novel in embedding community sectors within in-patient provision. Recruitment consisted of 15 purposefully sampled adult (i.e., ≥18 years) service users from across in-patient care and supported community living. The sample approximately reflected the demographics of the Service and comprised of ten men and five women. Twelve identified as white British, and three identified as being of ethnic minority origin/heritage. Their ages ranged from 18 to 60 years. Photo-elicitation was used to enrich data collection; semi-structured interviews were based around photographs taken by participants.

Case Study 6.2

The study (Taylor et al., 2020) included a total of 12 people, comprising nine women and three men who at the time were geographically located in the United Kingdom. Eight of them identified as being asylum-seekers and three had attained refugee status in the UK, and one participant chose not to disclose their status to the research team. The participants were of African (different countries) and Iranian heritage. Their ages ranged from 28 to 61 years. Length of stay in the United Kingdom ranged from 5 to 21 years. Participants undertook a two-stage interview process: stage one was focused around significant artefacts chosen by participants; stage two included a more general exploration of experiences of trauma.

Our first case study involved service users as research participants and was developed in a mental health service where the most prevalent diagnoses were made under the classification of psychotic disorders (Smith et al., 2021). Typical challenges experienced by those presenting with psychotic processes include confusion, perceiving things that others do not, holding strong beliefs that are not commonly shared, and emotional changes. Many service users are susceptible to multiple vulnerabilities because of their individual circumstances and/or previous trauma, including complex health and relational issues. In particular, ineffective and negative relationships can lead to isolation, a lack of trust, and feeling unsafe which can cause barriers to developing future positive relationships (Gilburt et al., 2008). Furthermore, service users or those accessing support/care services for psychological distress can often find themselves in a disempowered position where their rights to be involved in their own treatment and care are challenged (Rush, 2004). Developing positive connections with others can be attributed to finding our place in the world (Jacobson & Greenley, 2001) and promote safety and autonomy (Smith et al., 2021). As a result, these individuals require an approach to recovery and post-traumatic growth that appreciates and understands the value of reparative human connection.

The second case study involved refugees and asylum-seekers as research participants (Taylor et al., 2020). Refugees and asylum-seekers have a wide range of needs. Experiences of torture, trauma, and exile inevitably impact on their lives and disempower them personally and politically (Kenny et al., 2022). Many refugees and asylum-seekers who seek asylum in the USA or Europe have experienced or witnessed torture, war, sexual violence, stress, trauma, and multiple complex losses, and present with notifiable infectious diseases and dislocation from social networks, or families (Burnett & Peel, 2001; Satinsky et al., 2019). In addition to this, they also experience post-traumatic stress, generalised anxiety, depression, wounds of torture, destitution, and the need for advocacy and legal representation (Burnett & Peel, 2001; Satinsky et al., 2019; Taylor et al., 2020). As a result, clinical formulation and Eurocentric perspectives of trauma, must take account of cross-cultural sensitivity and difference. IPA, as a methodological approach, is congruent with the epistemological view that the lived experience of trauma is best understood from the perspective of *those who have lived it.*

Table 6.1 presents a synthesised table of themes drawn from both studies (Smith et al., 2021; Taylor et al., 2020), in order to illuminate a relational understanding of the lived experiences of both groups. This illustrates how findings mirror one another in relation to personal journeys of trauma, psychological distress, and towards recovery.

The journey for service users 'begins with *challenge* and moves towards making *connections* with others. Here *power* dynamics are often experienced and addressed in the development of a greater sense of *independence*. This then provides opportunities for raised *awareness* around the possibilities of recovery and a new-found *hope*' (Smith et al., 2021, p.1106). In comparison, the journey for asylum-seekers and refugees

Table 6.1 Summary of themes

Service users: Smith et al., 2021	Asylum-seekers: Taylor et al., 2020
CHALLENGE	STRUGGLE
Personal experiences	Struggle with legitimacy and not being believed
Relationships	Struggle with concealing emotions
Limitations in care	Struggle as a journey
Response to adversity	
Resilience	
CONNECTION	CONNECTION
Bonds	Interpersonal connections
Meaning from experiences	Importance of present connecting relationships in the face of loss/trauma
Attachments	Connecting to God/faith
Trauma	
POWER	LOSS
Control	Loss of predictability, stability, and security
Lack of choice	Loss of interpersonal connections
Relational dynamics	Loss of old identity and a sense of belonging
	Loss of dignity
INDEPENDENCE	PERCEIVED HELPFUL COPING STRATEGIES
Engagement	Gratitude
Self-agency	Helping others/giving service to others
Personal responsibility	Recognising identity shifts/personal growth
AWARENESS	MAKING SENSE OF MEMORY
Level of understanding	Impact of trauma on memory processes
Engagement with external perspectives	Importance of memory for recovery
HOPE	HOPE
Change	Getting back to real life
Insight	Religious faith/spirituality
Self-belief	Post-traumatic growth
Acceptance	Acceptance
Aspirations	

begins with the high level of trauma experienced by individuals that includes experiences of *loss*, the *struggle* faced by those forced to flee their homes, and the challenging experience of *making sense of memory*, which can be both a source of trauma and healing. Making *connections* through legal and support services, religion/spirituality, counselling/psychotherapy, and social support allows for movement towards developing *helpful coping strategies*. Support from others towards embracing an attitude of acceptance allows individuals to feel *hope* for a different future (see Taylor et al., 2020). Across both studies participants identify the fundamental role of connectedness for recovery and post-traumatic growth.

Challenge and *Struggle*

All participants spoke about personal *challenges* or *struggles* they experienced in relation to others. For service users, examples included difficulties experienced in relationships both within services and in the community, such as a lack of understanding and compassion, as well as limitations they had experienced in their care. One participant shared: *"I think if they hadn't feared for their jobs, if it wasn't illegal, they probably would have hit me, hurt me in some way"*. Asylum-seekers and refugees spoke of the struggle with legitimacy and not being believed by authorities, as well as having to conceal their emotions. For example, one participant said: *"I carried my pain. That's why I will say, I will smile while I'm bleeding inside… No one helped me"*. These experiences of challenge and struggle resulted in participants undergoing difficult psychological journeys that impacted on their ability to be in relationship with others. Thus, it is important that services maintain the trauma-informed position of 'what happened to you?' rather than 'what is wrong with you?' and extend an invitation to share the trauma narrative/experience, in order to know how best to meet an individual's needs.

Connection

Connection was a key theme shared across both studies. Service users spoke of the relationships and bonds they had made whilst in mental health services and the meaning they had made from their experiences with others. Meaningful connections were valued, as expressed by one participant: *"It is important to have people in your life"*, and also linked to enabling improvements in physical health, social functioning, and self-esteem. Asylum-seekers and refugees spoke on the importance of connecting to God/faith, experiencing kindness from others, and being of service to others in similar situations. One participant expressed: *"I wanted to do something that I know I can... It's for the refugees. I'm working as a volunteer, as an interpreter"*. Giving back to the community or to those in similar situations was seen as pivotal across both studies as this gave individuals a sense of agency and purpose. Hence, providing opportunities for a variety of relationships to develop within services enables enriching connection with others that is both meaningful and transforming.

Power and *Loss*

The participants all spoke in some way about their relationship with *power* and *loss*. For example, service users spoke of their challenging journey through mental health services where they experienced feeling powerless, particularly with regard to diagnosis, hospitalisation, and relational dynamics. One participant stated: "*...I definitely had a sense that my rights had been taken away from me...*". For refugees and asylum-seekers their lived experience and narrative nearly always started with experiencing trauma and loss of family, loss of home, and loss of connection. When speaking of the impact of this, one participant said: "*...I do not trust anymore. I've lost the trust...*". This experience of powerlessness and loss contributed to the psychological distress and breakdown of relationships. Thus, it is clear to see that any interventions, service settings, approaches to treatment, or support needs to be steeped in 'power-with' rather than 'power-over' and a trauma-informed approach which considers what has been lost and how that can be reintegrated.

Independence and *Perceived Helpful Coping Strategies*

All participants shared experiences of working towards gaining greater *independence* which included talking about *perceived helpful coping strategies*. Being supported by staff to engage in activities that improved their individual sense of wellness was highly valued by service users, as expressed here: *"I felt great after, just for my own mental health, going for a run, a short run"*. Perceived helpful coping strategies, as expressed by asylum-seekers and refugees, included becoming more accepting towards their situation and having gratitude towards those who showed them kindness, for example: "*…these people, they are doing their best. They are helping. Yes, I really appreciate that*". From both studies it is clear that opportunities that allow for positive engagement with self and others can result in increased agency and improved changes to self-concept. Services that promote such opportunities enable individuals to take more responsibility for their own journey towards post-traumatic growth, thus allowing for increased levels of self-confidence and resilience.

Awareness and *Making Sense of Memory*

Across both studies participants spoke of the importance of developing a greater *awareness* of self which involved *making sense of memory* of past trauma in order to become more familiar with their own journey towards post-traumatic growth. For service users this involves discussing coping mechanisms to gain perspective through developing self-awareness and making sense of past and current traumatic experiences, as evidenced here: "*I have heard quite a few people do actually listen to music and it helps them. Even people without mental health problems*". Asylum-seekers and refugees talked of the complications around the impact of trauma, including difficulties in memory recall, as explained by one participant: "*…I forget things a lot, because my head is full of problems*". Participants across both studies noted that accessing positive memories felt therapeutic and went some way towards alleviating painful experiences, both past and present. Thus, services that support those who wish to understand their experiences in more depth can help individuals move towards post-traumatic growth.

Hope

Embedded in all participants' narratives is the theme of *hope*, which was mainly represented by the changes participants had experienced by being in relationship with others. For service users, the experience of connecting with others offers hope that they can move away from difficult past experiences, for example: "*…this is like a whole new experience for me, like being ready to move on and having people supporting me*". Whilst asylum-seekers and refugees recognise that hope can be found in religious and spiritual connections, as well as in the knowledge that difficult situations can be transitory, as explained here: "*…I just keep telling myself it's going to end soon, and life goes on*". All participants spoke of the insights they had gained through relationships that have enabled a greater sense of self-belief and acceptance which has encouraged them to set future goals and aspirations. Thus, it is clear that enabling strong connections within services is an important step in supporting individuals move towards a more hopeful future.

Reconceptualising Relational Trauma and Recovery Through a Relational and Existential-Phenomenological Approach

Having presented the themes (Challenge, Struggle, Connection, Power, Loss, Independence, Perceived Helpful Coping Strategies, Awareness, Making Sense of Memory, Hope) conceptualised from the case studies (Smith et al., 2021; Taylor et al., 2020) we concur that these lived experiences directly speak to the world *as it is lived* from the perspective of *those who are living it*. Furthermore, it is evident that there are numerous pre- and post-traumatic sequelae, as well as multiple factors that may lead to psychological distress and complex trauma for people in both these groups. Additionally, we note that an effective conceptualisation of the multiple traumas they face should include a *culturally appropriate* relational-centred, existential-phenomenological approach. Given that the themes listed above convey relational trauma we assert that therapeutic working should be informed by a relational approach.

> *It's the relationship that heals, the relationship that heals, the relationship that heals…* (Yalom, 1989/2012, p. 112)

Relational trauma can leave a devastating impact on an individual's ability to develop and maintain positive relationships, as well as their mental health. Yalom (1989/2012) highlights the position we are advocating for when working in services supporting those experiencing trauma and psychological distress.

Relational-Centred Principles

In brief the key relational principles we refer to (Finlay, 2016; Paul & Charura, 2014), as applicable to this chapter include:

- We are born in and grow through relationships, and these relationships are of fundamental importance in the development of personality and a sense of self;
- Our personal problems arise in and through relationship;
- Our ability to resolve practical problems is often facilitated when we can access our own internal resources;
- We have a built-in propensity to grow to our full potential;
- We are social beings and without relationships we do not develop;
- We are part of a growthful and evolving universe.
- Basic assumptions for change and recovery (Charura & Smith, 2023; Finlay, 2016; Paul & Charura, 2014) through therapy/services are:
- The therapy/services offer a microcosm of the social world. The dynamics that emerge within therapy/services supporting people experiencing trauma may well mirror processes happening outside the therapeutic space and/or systemically;
- A *relational approach* endeavours to offer a space that is collaborative, compassionate, safe, secure, and containing of the trauma experiences;
- That the relationship or services offer the right conditions for healing, therapeutic engagement, transformation, or recovery;
- The therapeutic relationship and process is at the heart of this approach.

Alongside these principles it is important to have an awareness of the mutual impact that those accessing services and mental health professionals have on one another (transferential dynamics). This may emerge as a result of the impact of the wider systemic challenges that individuals presenting with trauma and psychological distress might have faced. It is also important to have an awareness of the diverse ways people may experience the impact of trauma and psychological distress, and how transformation or recovery might ensue. Furthermore, we must acknowledge the existential phenomenological challenges and difficulties in working with trauma, and that for some it might be a life's work.

Integrating an Existential-Phenomenological Approach

An existentially-orientated approach is focused on examining how each unique human experiences their way of being and continually attempts to understand their life's meaning (Finlay, 2016; van Deurzen, 2014). Alongside this, Yalom's (1980) assertion of the four givens of human existence: death, freedom, isolation, and meaninglessness, and how we confront these, offered us a good base to understand trauma and psychological distress from an existential-phenomenological approach as presented in this chapter. For example, these four givens of human existence impact all participants regardless of whether they are service users (Case Study 6.1) or asylum-seekers and refugees (Case Study 6.2).

An existential-phenomenological position is one where the practitioner engages with the individual's experience of trauma with genuine interest, curiosity, and care (Finlay, 2016). This aligns with Spinelli's (1997/2006, p. 5) perspective that existential-phenomenological theory offers us "a view of human existence that places anxiety at its centre". Furthermore, he argues that our experiences of living are "never certain, never fully predictable, never secure", and thus the very act of embracing life presents human beings with all manner of challenges which include, for example, what the aims and purposes of life/existence are and how we attach meaning to our experiences (Spinelli, 2006, p. 5). Thus, he asserts the existential-phenomenological lens can be understood as a clarification of the client's self-construct and "exploration of the client's way of being-in-the-world (and the contradictions, conflicts, and anxieties that these evoke or avoid) than it is about symptom removal 'ego strengthening', 'rational functioning', and so forth" (Spinelli, 2006, p. 5). Therefore, taking this approach befits working with the diversity of clients in different contexts and services and the focus can be, for example, on raising the client's awareness of their experiences, meanings, and needs in relation to the trauma and its presentation.

Working relationally and with an existential-phenomenological focused approach means engaging with the trauma/psychological presentation in the here-and-now, whilst acknowledging that each contact and intervention is idiosyncratic and thus must be attuned to each client's specific needs (Charura & Smith, 2023; DeYoung, 2003; Erskine, 2015; Finlay, 2016; Spinelli, 2015). The relationally-centred existential-phenomenological lens highlights the importance of being non-judgmental, open, empathic, and curious about the trauma (Finlay, 2016). It also requires openness and competence to work with the individual's experiences of relationships that have been severed, or indeed with the fragmentation, and/or violation of a significant relationship(s) or boundaries of self.

Recommendations for Working Through Relational Trauma

Having outlined, analysed, and conceptualised the different themes in relation to the case studies presented, we now conclude with recommendations for working with *relational trauma* in the context of services, interventions, and therapeutic encounters. In this case these are relational-centred existential-phenomenological approaches.

Our seven recommendations are for practitioners to:

1. Engage with an understanding of *relational trauma* from different perspectives (to include individual and social context), as well as taking a trauma-informed position of 'what happened to you?' rather than 'what is wrong with you?'.

2. Encourage those accessing services to seek opportunities for connection, for example, through collaboration with practitioners/service providers and the wider community.
3. Acknowledge the impact of inter/intra power relations between self, society, and within systems and how this can impact and perpetuate psychological distress/trauma.
4. Have an awareness and embodying approach of 'power-with' rather than 'power-over', as this 'power-with' stance facilitates recovery/reintegration.
5. Promote opportunities for those accessing services to build autonomy, independence, and to engage with helpful coping strategies whilst offering a supportive environment and professional therapeutic relationship.
6. Champion and integrate interventions that promote reflective practice relating to experiencing trauma and life events which contributed to psychological disintegration/maladjustment/dis-ease.
7. Offer a relational frame which embodies a contemporary understanding of *relational trauma* and commits to a therapeutic approach where the facilitated conditions optimise capacity for relational connections and reintegration of the fragmented parts of self/self-concept/self-structure and/or the psyche.

In concluding we note that this chapter illuminates not only the power of IPA as a methodology in engaging with the lived experience in different individuals and context but also how practitioners can integrate diversity and philosophical approaches within *relational trauma* work.

Acknowledgements The research presented in this chapter was funded by Leeds and York Partnership NHS Foundation Trust and NHS Leeds North Clinical Commissioning Group (Case Study 6.1) and Leeds Beckett University (Case Study 6.2).

References

American Psychological Association. (2022). *Trauma.* Available at: https://www.apa.org/topics/trauma

Brocki, J. M., & Wearden, A. J. (2006). A critical evaluation of the use of interpretative phenomenological analysis (IPA) in health psychology. *Psychology and Health, 21*(1), 87–108. https://doi.org/10.1080/14768320500230185

Burnett, A., & Peel, M. (2001). Asylum seekers and refugees in Britain: The health of survivors of torture and organised violence. *BMJ: British Medical Journal, 322*(7286), 606–609. https://doi.org/10.1136/bmj.322.7286.606

Charura, D., & Smith, P. (2023). Post-traumatic stress disorder. In C. Feltham, T. Hanley, & L. A. Winter (Eds.), *The SAGE handbook of counselling and psychotherapy* (5th ed.). Sage.

Cloitre, M., Courtois, C. A., Charuvastra, A., Carapezza, R., Stolbach, B. C., & Green, B. L. (2011). Treatment of complex PTSD: Results of the ISTSS expert clinician survey on best practices. *Journal of Traumatic Stress, 24*, 615–627. https://doi.org/10.1002/jts.20697

Cooper, M. (2007). Humanizing psychotherapy. *Journal of Contemporary Psychotherapy, 37*(1), 11–16.

DeYoung, P. A. (2003). *Relational psychotherapy: A primer.* Brunner-Routledge.

Erskine, R. G. (2015). *Relational patterns, therapeutic presence: Concepts and practice of integrative psychotherapy.* Karnac.

Farina, B., Liotti, M., & Imperatori, C. (2019). The role of attachment trauma and disintegrative pathogenic processes in the traumatic-dissociative dimension. *Frontiers in Psychology, 10*, 933. https://doi.org/10.3389/fpsyg.2019.00933

Finlay, L. (2016). *Relational integrative psychotherapy: Processes and theory in practice.* Wiley.

Gilburt, H., Rose, D., & Slade, M. (2008). The importance of relationships in mental health care: A qualitative study of service users' experiences of psychiatric hospital admission in the UK. *BMC Health Services Research, 8*(1), 92.

Isobel, S., Goodyear, M., & Foster, K. (2017). Psychological trauma in the context of familial relationships: A concept analysis. *Trauma Violence Abuse, 1524838017726424.* https://doi.org/10.1177/1524838017726424

Jacobson, N., & Greenley, D. (2001). What is recovery? A conceptual model and explication. *Psychiatric Services, 52*(4), 482–485. https://doi.org/10.1176/appi.ps.52.4.482

Kenny, M. A., Grech, C., & Procter, N. (2022). A trauma informed response to COVID 19 and the deteriorating mental health of refugees and asylum seekers with insecure status in Australia. *International Journal of Mental Health Nursing, 31*(1), 62–69. https://doi.org/10.1111/inm.12932

Lachal, J., Speranza, M., Taieb, O., Falissard, B., Lefevre, H., Moro, M. R., & Revah-Levy, A. (2012). Qualitative research using photo-elicitation to explore the role of food in family relationships among obese adolescents. *Appetite, 58*(3), 1099–1105.

Paul, S., & Charura, D. (2014). *An introduction to the therapeutic relationship in counselling and psychotherapy*. Sage.

Rush, B. (2004). Mental health service user involvement in England: Lessons from history. *Journal of Psychiatric and Mental Health Nursing, 11*(3), 313–318. https://doi.org/10.1111/j.1365-2850.2004.00728.x

Sar, V. (2011). Developmental trauma, complex PTSD, and the current proposal of DSM-5. *European Journal of Psychotraumatology, 2*, 1. https://doi.org/10.3402/ejpt.v2i0.5622

Satinsky, E., Fuhr, D. C., Woodward, A., Sondorp, E., & Roberts, B. (2019). Mental health care utilisation and access among refugees and asylum seekers in Europe: A systematic review. *Health Policy, 123*(9), 851–863. https://doi.org/10.1016/j.healthpol.2019.02.007

Shaw, R. (2010). Embedding reflexivity within experiential qualitative psychology. *Qualitative Research in Psychology, 7*(3), 233–243. https://doi.org/10.1080/14780880802699092

Smith, J. A., & Osborn, M. (2008). Interpretative phenomenological analysis. In J. A. Smith (Ed.), *Qualitative psychology: A practical guide to methods* (2nd ed., pp. 53–80). Sage.

Smith, J. A., Flowers, P., & Larkin, M. (2009). *Interpretative phenomenological analysis: Theory, method and research*. Sage.

Smith, P., Simpson, L., & Madill, A. (2021). Service user experiences of a novel in-reach rehabilitation and recovery service for people with profound and enduring mental health needs. *International Journal of Mental Health Nursing, 30*(5), 1106–1116. https://doi.org/10.1111/inm.12861

Smith, J. A., Flowers, P., & Larkin, M. (2022). *Interpretative phenomenological analysis: Theory, method and research* (2nd ed.). Sage.

Spinelli, E. (1997/2006). *Tales of un-knowing. Therapeutic encounters from an existential perspective*. PCCS Books.

Spinelli, E. (2015). *Practicing existential therapy: The relational world* (2nd ed.).

Taylor, S., Charura, D., Williams, G., Shaw, M., Allan, J., Cohen, E., Meth, F., & O'Dwyer, L. (2020). An interpretative phenomenological analysis of the lived experiences of trauma among a sample of asylum seekers and refugees. *Traumatology*. https://doi.org/10.1037/trm0000250

Terock, J., Van der Auwera, S., Janowitz, D., Spitzer, C., Barnow, S., Miertsch, M., Freyberger, H. J., & Grabe, H. J. (2016). From childhood trauma to adult dissociation: The role of PTSD and alexithymia. *Journal of Anxiety Disorders, 49*, 374–382. https://doi.org/10.1159/000449004

van der Kolk, B. A. (1996). The complexity of adaptation to trauma: Self-regulation, stimulus discrimination and characterological development. In B. A. van der Kolk, A. C. McFarlane, & L. Weisaeth (Eds.), *Traumatic stress: The effects of overwhelming experience on mind, body, and society* (pp. 182–213). Guilford Press.

van der Kolk, B. (2014). *The body keeps the score: Mind, brain and body in the transformation of trauma*. Penguin.

van Deurzen, E. (2012). *Existential counselling and psychotherapy in practice*. Sage.

van Deurzen, E. (2014). *Existential psychotherapy and counselling in practice* (3rd ed.). Sage.

Williamson, V., Creswell, C., Fearon, P., Hiller, R. M., Walker, J., & Halligan, S. L. (2017). The role of parenting behaviors in childhood post-traumatic stress disorder: A meta-analytic review. *Clinical Psychology Review, 53*, 1–13. https://doi.org/10.1016/j.cpr.2017.01.005

Yalom, I. D. (1980). *Existential psychotherapy*. Basic Books.

Yalom, I. D. (1989/2012). *Love's executioner and other tales of psychotherapy*. Basic Books.

Part III

Peers, Family and Community: Care and Companionship Through Distress and Recovery

7

Understanding the Value Base That Supports the Development of Peer Support Relationships

Humma Andleeb, Richard Currie, Fozia Haider, Raj Hazzard, Tanya Mackay, Andreja Mesarič, Jennie Parker, Vanessa Pinfold, Laura Richmond, and Rose Thompson

What Is Peer Support?

The term peer support is used to describe the kind of support that people may offer one another when they share and support each other through similar (often difficult or traumatic) experiences (Mead & MacNeil, 2006; Repper & Carter, 2010). Examples include groups of new mothers, groups for people with long-term physical health conditions, or

H. Andleeb
UCL, London, UK

R. Hazzard • T. Mackay (✉) • V. Pinfold • R. Thompson (✉)
McPin Foundation, London, UK
e-mail: rosethompson@mcpin.org

R. Currie • F. Haider • A. Mesarič
Independent, London, UK

Z. Boden-Stuart, M. Larkin (eds.), *Relationships and Mental Health*,
https://doi.org/10.1007/978-3-031-50047-3_7

long-running projects such as Alcoholics Anonymous (Watson & Meddings, 2019). In a mental health context, 'peer support' describes the kind of support that people who have experienced similar mental health challenges may offer one another. This occurs in a wide variety of settings, from informal conversations between friends or acquaintances through to structured formal conversations taking place within mental health services provided by employed peer support workers (Adame & Leitner, 2008; Lloyd-Evans et al., 2014).

All of the authors on this chapter have worked with the McPin Foundation either as peer researchers who had lived experience of peer support in a mental health context, as researchers who had worked on research or evaluation projects related to peer support happening in a mental health services or mental health in community settings, or as managers who had project managed those projects and had line managed peer researchers in that context. This chapter is based on the knowledge acquired through seven years' worth of experience working on a range of research and evaluation projects in different peer support settings (between 2015 and 2022). In writing this chapter, two of the researchers named above took on the bulk of the writing, based on the work we have produced throughout that time, and the remaining authors commented on the draft from their specific perspectives. However, that initial draft was deeply informed by the conversations and ideas that all of the authors listed above have contributed across those seven years to different projects, and thus all should be considered as taking an essential role in producing the ideas that form the basis of this chapter. The authors of this chapter have been listed in alphabetical order to reflect this.

One of our researchers, who is also a disability activist with lived experience of being a peer supporter, reflected that he sees peer support as a continuum of practices that includes both very informal and formal structured practices within its range. There are also a variety of

J. Parker
Berkshire Healthcare NHS Foundation Trust, Berkshire, UK

L. Richmond
Department of Clinical, Educational and Health Psychology, UCL, London, UK

terminologies used for people in peer support roles, including peer supporters, peer worker and peer support workers (Vaughn et al., 2018). In this chapter, we will focus on the kind of peer support that commonly happens in a community setting, underpinned by a more informal ethos, often hosted by organisations from the voluntary, community and social enterprise (VCSE) sector.

Evolution of Peer Support in the Global North

Peer support amongst people experiencing mental health challenges has a long history, emerging out of political movements responding to clinical practices that felt harmful, including restraint, seclusion and coercion (Mead & Macneil, 2006; Noorani, 2013; Pelletier & Davidson, 2015). As a result, peer support emerging out of this movement was deliberately non-clinical and organically developed to offer an alternative approach of mutual support for and by people who shared mental health challenges (Faulkner & Kalathil, 2012). Over time this approach has grown in popularity and has been adopted by many groups and organisations who are not grounded in this original political discourse. Notably, there is an increasing momentum to embed peer support workers across statutory services (NHS Mental Health Implementation Plan, 2019).

This is important to consider when exploring peer support in the current mental health landscape, as it has resulted in a diversity of views about what constitutes 'good' peer support, and which applications may or may not be acceptable. For example, there is a wide range of conflicting views on the implementation of peer support within clinical services, and the extent to which this represents the institutionalisation of peer support, or a positive development in mental health care. Gillard (2019) surmised that the research on peer support provided by peer workers tends to describe interventions that align with a medical model and suggests that peer workers within statutory services may be tasked with delivering support that is based on an illness management approach whilst working in 'para-clinical roles'. This involves identifying 'what is wrong' with an individual and working with a peer worker with the overall aim of promoting 'recovery' (itself a contested concept, see Woods et al., 2019). This approach can be seen as being in direct conflict with the political history of peer support as a holistic community-based alternative to clinical care (Mead & MacNeil, 2006; Faulkner & Basset 2012). Some authors within mental health and disability activism communities have strong concerns that this activity represents the co-option of both peer support and the concept of recovery by systems that have been viewed as oppressive (Beresford & Russo, 2016). Further, people have raised concerns that the professionalisation of peer support roles in the statutory setting may homogenise experiential knowledge, risking the loss of core values regarding equality and mutuality (Beresford & Russo, 2016; Faulkner & Basset 2012; Woods et al., 2019). However, it is important to note that for some people, there is a sense of safety associated with more formal clinical peer support structures, including in the maternal mental health context (Mackay et al., 2022). In these contexts, the challenge may be around communicating the special value and skills of peer support workers to some clinicians who are unfamiliar with its benefits (Wood, 2020). Further, one of our authors reflected that some people find peer support to be a useful complement to medical approaches that can form a distinct aspect of how they manage the mental health challenges that they face.

Peer support in the community tends to accommodate a greater range of approaches to distress and mental health challenges beyond the medical model. Here it is common for groups of people to come together to support each other and in doing so, to build communities in which peers consider one another to be equals, without the power imbalances that are inherent in professional or clinical roles. Peers are able to share stories and experiences, good and bad, and explore what may help, without potential interference from a clinical context in which experiences are pathologised.

One of the most notable features we have observed of peer support in community settings is the diversity of contexts and styles in which it can be found (Mackay et al., 2022). In our work across numerous community peer support projects, we encountered three main models: groups, one-to-one forms such as peer mentoring or befriending, and online via digital platforms (The Side by Side Research Consortium, 2017). Some projects blended aspects of the different models together or brought in additional features such as support from clinical services (Mind & The McPin Foundation, 2019a, b). This demonstrates the flexibility of the peer support model, which can be adapted to suit different physical or virtual contexts, and the particular needs of different groups of people. However, whilst there is great diversity amongst model(s) and contexts of peer support, the relationships that form tend to be similar in nature.

Personal Reflection on Peer Support by RH—Peer Friendships Undress Emotions

This is a kind of friendship that finds itself. Someone with whom you can be your vulnerable, unfiltered self and be accepted for it. It is a space where un-common experiences you've had—ones that summon pain and deep-rooted emotions—get a chance to come to the surface and be shared. Often [these are] ones shrouded in shame, unprocessed grief and a healthy dose of self-pity. It's those rare friendships where you get to go deep, and the other person is not scared off. They meet you right in the darkness and validate it, not because they have been trained that this is the right thing to do, but because they too have felt the darkness and sense it is the right thing to do. In my experiences, these friendships are rare, but they secure the soul like no other. I leave this kind of moment with renewed confidence and hope.

The Peer Support Relationship

Within the academic and grey literature, and across our work with a variety of different projects, we have found that the nature of the peer support relationship tends to be described in similar ways with some typical characteristics. These are encapsulated by the activities people do together, and how they engage in those activities. Across the literature, different terms may have been employed to describe the characteristics below. These include:

Sharing Experiences of Mental Health Challenges

The core activity that peer relationships are often built around is sharing similar experiences of mental health challenges with one another (Faulkner & Basset, 2012). Individuals may choose to do this to a greater or lesser extent at different times, and different groups of people may use different language. However, the sharing is reciprocal in nature as everyone involved has the opportunity to share their own experiences and learn from the experiences of others. Experiences directly around mental health can be difficult to articulate, and the knowledge that people are talking to one another based on some shared understanding can enable others to feel heard and understood. Being able to talk with others who may 'have been there' and have an intrinsic understanding and empathy based on that experience, rather than trying to explain themselves to people who 'have not been there', can be a huge relief and the starting point to reparation. One of our authors reflected that:

> *Understanding from reading about something or from practising as a clinician is a sort of understanding, but it's a different sort to the understanding that comes from living through something.*

However, as noted by Faulkner and Kalathil (2012), experience of mental health difficulties alone may not be 'enough' for a group of people to recognise one another as peers. In some contexts, other personal characteristics and life experiences may also be essential, such as culture, disability, racialised identities, sexuality, or traumatic experiences.

Taking an Interest in One Another's 'Whole Lives'

Peer support relationships usually begin with people getting to know one another, often based on sharing experiences about what has happened to them and what they may have learned through that process. This process often includes peers talking about their lives in a way that extends beyond their experiences with mental health, to include aspects of themselves and their journey that are essential to understanding them as a person. With careful thought, peer support can be incorporated into trauma-informed approaches that prioritise storytelling, in that it makes space for people to share their stories safely and without judgement (Blanch et al., 2012; Mackay et al., 2022). This can be helpful in reducing stigma, and for some individuals, it may be the only acceptable form of support. This may be an outcome of a range of factors, including cultural or family perspectives on mental health, previous experiences with statutory services, or the availability of appropriate local clinical services. Some participants in our evaluation of the Side by Side project (Side by Side Research Consortium, 2017) talked about the natural warmth or 'realness' of the interactions that happen in community peer support in the absence of clinical boundaries.

Considering One Another to Be Equals

People in peer support relationships consider one another to be equals. They recognise that each person has valuable insight and expertise about managing mental health challenges based on their own experiences, without the need for formal, 'book learned' qualifications. This also means that peers share power and responsibility within more formal or structured peer support settings. This may mean that different people take responsibility for different aspects of the peer support at different times (examples include leading structured conversations, arranging venues or organising refreshments). When an individual chooses to take on or give up responsibilities may be influenced by what that individual may be feeling or experiencing at a given time and what other events may be happening in their lives.

Boundaries

In more structured or formal settings, peers typically co-design a set of 'ground rules' within which they all agree to participate. As projects progress and others join, peers usually have the opportunity to review and discuss what the ground rules of a space may be, and to agree on changes as required to ensure the safety and comfort of all. A key aspect of the process of setting ground rules is that this is done mutually among peers. Everyone has the opportunity to contribute to the discussion around what ground rules should be, and this process may be repeated over time. In many projects, peers also take mutual responsibility for acting within these boundaries, and in deciding how to respond if someone is felt to be acting outside of them in ways that do not feel safe to other peers (Side by Side Consortium, 2017). In more informal settings, boundaries exist but may be arrived at through less clearly articulated processes.

Pooling Expertise Based on Lived Experience

Peers recognise each other as bringing invaluable experiential knowledge and expertise that can be helpful both to other peers as individuals and to our collective understanding of mental health (Faulkner & Basset, 2012). Faulkner and Basset (2012) have noted that "others who have had similar experiences may be able to shed light on your own, can offer genuine empathy, new insights and potentially also shared strategies for managing particular difficulties" (p. 54). It can be validating to hear peers share their stories and find that these are heard and valued by others around them. This can be a source of encouragement and support and can inspire people to open up and share their own stories, particularly those experiences which might be associated with shame or other painful feelings.

Has a Different Feel to the Relationships Peers May Have with Friends or Family

Peers may feel more comfortable sharing their experiences with other peers than with family members or friends. One of our authors who has participated in peer support reflected that sharing these kinds of problems with friends or family involves a lot of emotional labour, balancing the need to avoid causing distress with making themselves feel understood. This emotional labour may be far less pronounced in a peer relationship where both parties have a baseline understanding of the difficulties involved. Another author reflected that there can be history or baggage attached to our close relationships that may complicate these conversations that peer relationships don't have.

Not Time-Limited

Community peer support is typically available for peers to dip in and out of for as long as a project is running, and in informal setting, this may continue indefinitely. This allows relationships to form that are organic and natural, as they can unfold over time with mutual experiences.

Personal Reflection by RH—Peer Groups Collect Power

The peer groups I have joined have been voluntary, meeting around a more specific set of experiences. For me, these are 'other' spaces for experiences that I felt 'othered' by. This is somewhat mirrored in the discrete nature of group names, advertising their purpose behind symbols and metaphors. At first, I have found groups awkward, like a party where everyone is supposed to know each other but where in reality we are all strangers. The distance dissolves as people begin to share stories. I have learnt and grown much from this kind of sharing. Sharing can make visible 'hidden in plain sight' experiences, those that are sometimes invisible to the self because they are buried deep down. Stubborn beliefs and thought monsters become unveiled for what they are and this can sometimes lead to shifts in personal perspective. There is also a sense of collective power when taboo subjects get normalised. This solidarity can hop over into daily life. Sometimes I have worn it as a shield of armour when discrimination or assumptions come knocking. I have also taken the sense of solidarity and sharing wider, actively challenging perceptions out 'there'. For me, this type of leap to activism has been an important part of peer support.

Benefits of Peer Support

In their report, 'The freedom to be, the chance to dream', Faulkner and Kalathil (2012) cite the benefits of peer support as including personal, practical and social benefits for peers. The personal benefits they cited for everyone involved in peer support included confidence, self-esteem, companionship and empowerment. Practical benefits included accessing new information and locating other sources of support. Social benefits included feeling more integrated into the community, challenging stigma and discrimination, and being more accessible to people from specific marginalised groups.

Reflection by Richard Currie, Disability Activist and Peer Researcher

For me one of the most powerful things about peer support is empowerment, both from a personal and professional perspective. I have undertaken peer support roles in a number of informal and formal settings, and feel that the two forms of peer support have played a vital role in my development as an academic, an activist, and as a friend. It's about recognising and valuing other people's experiences. These experiences have given me the tools to draw on my lived experience effectively and sensitively in many circumstances where it could help other people.

What Is the Value Base That Underpins This Relationship?

Numerous organisations within the VCSE sector have created peer support charters and value sets that they consider to define what underpins the peer support relationship. Faulkner (2020) found that 'Shared Experience', 'Choice and Control', 'Mutuality', 'Reciprocity', 'Safety', 'Hope' and 'Empowerment' were values that had been identified across all forms of peer support.

In our own research on the values underpinning peer support, we have gathered data across several peer support projects, including interviewing numerous people who have been engaged in more organised forms of peer support (see Mackay et al., 2022; Side by Side Research Consortium, 2017).

In the first large evaluation we conducted we developed a value model that included six multifaceted values:

1. *Experience in Common*—Peers have experiences in common that are critical to recognising each other as peers. In a mental health context, this can mean experiences of mental health challenges, and/or social and emotional distress. In some contexts, this may also include additional aspects of identity such as gender, ethnicity or sexuality.
2. *Safety*—For peer support relationships to develop, they need to happen in a context that peers agree is both physically and emotionally safe. To achieve this, peers may mutually agree a set of 'ground rules'

for how to interact with one another, and the physical environment in which they meet must feel safe and be accessible.

3. *Choice and Control*—Individual peers are able to decide when and how they participate in peer support, how much they do or do not choose to share, and when and how they choose to share aspects of their story.
4. *Two-way Interactions*—Interactions in peer support involve the giving and receiving of support, whilst recognising that peers may give and receive more or less support at different times and in different contexts. This may be called reciprocity or mutuality in other frameworks.
5. *Human Connection*—Peers actively acknowledge that their connection with each other is based on experiences in common. They work together to create a warm, welcoming, friendly environment for all peers, and act with intentional kindness to one another. Peers understand and care for each other, creating a culture of companionship and belonging.
6. *Freedom to be Oneself*—Peers are able to express themselves freely without fear of judgement or the need to hide important aspects of their identities, and they are able to discuss difficult or painful topics with one another (Fig. 7.1).

These values were conceptualised as fitting together in a pyramid, so that three foundational base values ('Experience in Common', 'Choice and Control' and 'Safety') need to be in place within a peer support context to support the upper layers of the pyramid (on the second layer 'Two-way Interactions' and 'Human Connection', followed by 'Freedom to be Oneself' on the third layer).

Through our work on later evaluations, we found that it was necessary to modify the value sets depending on the specific setting. For example, in an evaluation of a large women-specific project conducted using trauma-informed principles, we adapted the foundation of the pyramid to include 'Trust' as one of the three foundational components, while 'Experience in Common' floated above these components as an intermediate layer supporting the same upper half of the pyramid. Taking a similar approach in a project specifically about peer support in a maternal

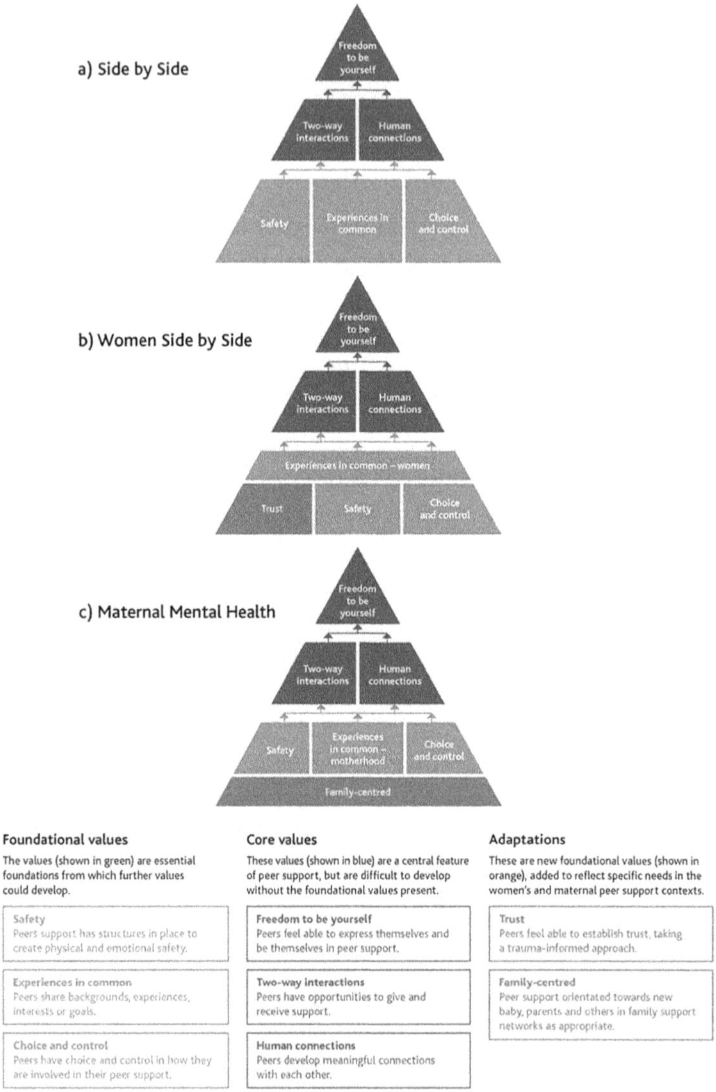

Fig. 7.1 Value pyramids produced from three different evaluations of Peer Support projects based in the community. (Mackay et al., 2022)

mental health context, we included a new foundational layer at the bottom to represent a 'Family-Centred' approach.

Through these three programmes of research, it became clear that the main set of values remained the same, with additions that were designed to adapt specifically to context. This principle also applies to how peer support may be organised in practice. Peers involved in different projects may make different decisions about how the above values are enacted, in order to create an environment in which the peer support relationship can flourish with specific groups of people and in different environments.

Reflection: Humma

It is apparent that peer support values are adapted and made relevant by the context of the groups. It feels like for me that values envision what is lacking in other services that may be made available to help people, which becomes fundamental within peer support where peers have the power to create their own rules to ensure peer support benefits them. The flexibility of peer support allows peers to shape and construct groups to suit their needs. Little to no other interventions offer similar flexibility to peer support. For me, this flexibility is key to making peer support a success and an ongoing benefit for peers.

How Do You Create the Conditions in Which Those Relationships Can Flourish?

Throughout our work across a number of projects, and within the literature, we found that people involved in peer support make a number of key decisions on how their projects are structured and organised to promote the development of context-dependent peer relationships (from Side by Side Research Consortium, 2017):

Facilitation

Many peer support projects adopt a structured approach to facilitation, in which the 'facilitator' is a specific (and often paid) role adopted by one individual with a specific set of responsibilities. Such responsibilities may include guiding structured conversations in a peer support group, and admin tasks relating to the running of a project and management of the space/venue. However, not all projects operate in this way: there are many projects in which these responsibilities are instead shared out or rotated amongst peers to enable everyone to be collectively responsible for group activities. We have encountered a range of different opinions around how important a facilitator is in peer support. Some individuals believe that a formalised facilitation role is essential to maintaining the safety of the group, while others feel it contradicts the ethos of all peers being equal together. It is likely that the facilitator role may be different in different contexts, for example in peer support for parents who may bring babies or toddlers with them, responsibilities may include ensuring there are changing facilities and toys available in the venue, along with managing any safeguarding concerns.

Types of Leadership

The prevailing view is that peer support should be led by peers, and that holistic support led by people without relevant lived experience, while also valuable, is not truly 'peer' support. However, in two of our research programmes, which were concerned with trauma-informed women's mental health peer support and maternal mental health peer support, both peers and people leading projects were explicit about their desire for input from clinicians into their project and for guidance that would assure the quality of peer support delivery, in one case resulting in the development of a new 'quality assurance framework' (Mackay et al., 2022). This can be viewed as a challenge to the view that all peer support should be solely peer-led and peer-run, if some peers themselves request clinical input. However, across all peer support contexts we have explored, there is a consistent belief that there must be peer involvement in how the peer support is set up and run, even where there is a non-peer in facilitative or leadership roles.

Focus of Peer Support Sessions

Across our work we have encountered great diversity in the types of activities that people may do together in peer support. These can range from more informal settings in which people sit and share stories or experiences through to structured activities such as guided walks, art or cookery lessons. In some projects, we found peer support organised in the context of training or educational sessions to occur alongside or during those activities.

Membership Type

We have identified a range of ways in which people who organise peer support groups define who can and cannot join. While all projects were shaped around some form of shared lived experience, the extent to which this experience was specified varied. Some groups were open to anyone with an experience of a mental health difficulty, while others were exclusively for specific groups of people defined by diagnosis or other aspects of their identity (for example, women-only spaces in the context of domestic abuse, or spaces for people who experience racism). How narrowly or broadly are the boundaries drawn around who can join has importance for the safety component of all the pyramids and also has implications for the accessibility of peer support for people who may not feel safe to express themselves in more general settings.

Organisational Support

In our work, we found that peer support projects were supported in a range of different ways. This included support from large local or national organisations who may supply funds and additional support like pre-existing ground rule templates and training, supervision and recruitment of facilitators. Other projects took a much more grassroots approach, were unfunded and self-organising, and frequently agreed amongst themselves how they would like to operate.

Paid Versus *Unpaid Roles*

There has been a much debate amongst the peer support community about the impact of paying people to do peer support roles. On the one hand, there is the argument that paying people for their work, which in these settings may take the form of administrative and logistical responsibilities, and as well as emotional labour, is important. Not providing payment may make these roles less accessible for those who do not have the financial and energetic resources to take on voluntary work. In many voluntary sector organisations, a group facilitator may be paid to support a group and take responsibility for its organisation. On the other hand, some have argued that paying peer supporters to support non-paid 'clients' creates an unhelpful power dynamic and contradicts the core principles of peer support.

Conclusion

Peer support can offer people who experience mental health challenges a valuable alternative or complementary form of support to that which may be offered through clinical services. It is a highly flexible form of support that is focussed on the relationship peers form with one another, defined within each particular peer relationship and context. In order for these relationships to flourish and to be sustainable, peer support values must translate into the practical decisions made during design and delivery of peer support. Decisions about how a peer support is organised in a particular setting will have an impact on the extent to which these relationships can develop and may involve thinking about; forms of leadership and facilitation; what the focus may be and who the peer support is for; ground rules; and practical considerations about the physical or online setting and administration. These decisions need to be carefully tailored to, and developed in collaboration with, the group of peers involved.

References

Adame, A., & Leitner, L. (2008). Breaking out of the mainstream: The evolution of peer support alternatives to the mental health system. *Ethical Human Psychology and Psychiatry, 10*(3), 146–162. https://doi.org/10.1891/1559-4343.10.3.146

Beresford, P., & Russo, J. (2016). Supporting the sustainability of Mad studies and preventing its co-option. *Disability & Society, 31*(2), 270–274. https://doi.org/10.1080/09687599.2016.1145380

Blanch, A., Filson, B., Penney, D., & Cave, C. (2012). *Engaging women in trauma-informed peer support: A guidebook.* Center for Mental Health Services, National Centre for Trauma-Informed Care. Available at: https://www.nasmhpd.org/sites/default/files/PeerEngagementGuide_Color_REVISED_10_2012.pdf

Faulkner, A. (2020). *The inconvenient complications of peer support: Part 1 & 2, National Survivor User Network.* Available from: https://www.nsun.org.uk/Blog/the-inconvenient-complications-of-peer-support & https://www.nsun.org.uk/blog/the-inconvenient-complications-of-peer-support-part-2

Faulkner, A., & Basset, T. (2012). A long and honourable history. *The Journal of Mental Health Training, Education and Practice, 7*(2), 53–59.

Faulkner, A., & Kalathil, J. (2012). *'The freedom to be, the chance to dream': Preserving user-led peer support in mental health.* Together.

Gillard, S. (2019). Peer support in mental health services: Where is the research taking us, and do we want to go there? *Journal of Mental Health, 28*(4), 341–344. https://doi.org/10.1080/09638237.2019.1608935

Lloyd-Evans, B., Mayo-Wilson, E., Harrison, B., et al. (2014). A systematic review and meta-analysis of randomised controlled trials of peer support for people with severe mental illness. *BMC Psychiatry 14*, 39. https://doi.org/10.1186/1471-244X-14-39

Mackay, T., Ahmed, N., Andleeb, H., Billsborough, J., Currie, R., Hazzard, R., Haider, F., Iqbal, N., Matthews, F., Mesarič, A., Parker, J., Pinfold, V., Richmond, L., Robotham, D., & Thompson, R. (2022). The evolution of community peer support values: Reflections from three UK mental health project teams. *Advances in Mental Health, 20*, 157. https://doi.org/10.1080/18387357.2022.2033128

Mead, S., & MacNeil, C. (2006). Peer support: What makes it unique? *International Journal of Psychosocial Rehabilitation, 10*(2), 29–37.

Mind & The McPin Foundation. (2019a). *Five principles for perinatal peer support.* Available at: https://maternalmentalhealthalliance.org/wp-content/uploads/mind-mcpin-perinatal-peer-support-principles-full-mmha-WEB.pdf

Mind & The McPin Foundation. (2019b). *Peer support principles for maternal mental health project.* Available at: https://mcpin.org/wp-content/uploads/2019/12/Peer-Support-Principles-for-perinatal-mental-Health-2019-FINAL.pdf

NHS Mental Health Implementation Plan. (2019). 2019/20 – 2023/24. NHS England. https://www.england.nhs.uk/publication/nhs-mental-health-implementation-plan-2019-20-2023-24/

Noorani, T. (2013). Service User Involvement, Authority and the 'Expert-by-Experience' in Mental Health. *Journal of Political Power, 6*(1), 49–68. https://doi.org/10.1080/2158379X.2013.774979

Pelletier, J. F., & Davidson, L. (2015). At the very roots of psychiatry as a new medical speciality: The Pinel-Pussin partnership. *Santé Mentale au Québec, 40*(1), 19–33.

Repper, J., & Carter, T. (2010). *Using personal experience to support others with similar difficulties: A review of literature on peer support in mental health services.* University of Nottingham & Together.

Side by Side Research Consortium. (2017). *Side by side: Early research findings.* Mind. Available at: https://mcpin.org/wp-content/uploads/Mind-Side-by-Side_Early-Research-findings.pdf

Vaughn, L. M., Whetstone, C., Boards, A., Busch, M. D., Magnusson, M., & Määttä, S. (2018). Partnering with insiders: A review of peer models across community-engaged research, education and social care. *Health & Social Care in the Community, 26*, 769–786. https://doi.org/10.1111/hsc.12562

Watson, E., & Meddings, S. (Eds.). (2019). *Peer support in mental health.* Bloomsbury: Red Globe Press.

Wood, L. (2020). *Peer workers in NHS perinatal mental health services: A values-based approach.* Mind. Available at: https://www.longtermplan.nhs.uk/wp-content/uploads/2019/07/nhs-mental-health-implementation-plan-2019-20-2023-24.pdf

Woods, A., Hart, A., & Spandler, H. (2019). The recovery narrative: Politics and possibilities of a genre. *Culture, Medicine, and Psychiatry, 46*, 221. https://doi.org/10.1007/s11013-019-09623-y

8

Exploring Family Experiences and Relationship Dynamics Where One Member Experiences Psychosis: *"We've Been on That Journey Together"*

Charlotte Marriott, Mark Bernard, and Michael Larkin

For young adults experiencing psychosis,[1] developmental milestones—such as leaving the familial environment, living independently and beginning to form their own social circles—are frequently delayed or disrupted (Harrop & Trower, 2001; Jungbauer et al., 2004). Families increasingly assume the responsibility for supporting the recovery of loved ones with severe mental illness. Professionals and services thus require strategies for effectively supporting family members. Such strategies require evidence about families' experiences, capabilities and needs in these situations.

[1] Psychosis is an umbrella term used to describe difficulties related to experiences of hallucinations, delusions, cognitive, social and emotional difficulties. This can manifest as a stand-alone episode; however, persistent difficulties may attract diagnoses of schizophrenia, schizo-affective disorder, post-partum psychosis, bipolar disorder, drug-induced psychosis, etc.

C. Marriott • M. Bernard
Birmingham Early Intervention in Psychosis Service, Birmingham, UK

M. Larkin (✉)
Aston University, Birmingham, UK
e-mail: m.larkin@aston.ac.uk

Z. Boden-Stuart, M. Larkin (eds.), *Relationships and Mental Health*,
https://doi.org/10.1007/978-3-031-50047-3_8

A review by Saunders (2003) reported that coping strategies, caregiver burden, resiliency, depression, social support, behavioural difficulties and family functioning were the primary focus and outcome of research on this topic. Saunders described family adjustment and adaptation as the key constructs in crisis management. Where family *relationships* were discussed, it was regarding how parental expressed emotion impacted upon the patient's symptomology, burden and mental wellbeing. Saunders noted that employment, finances, marital relationships and physical health permanently affected the family's identity, roles and relationships. Within the review, these latter issues were only briefly identified (by a single article written over 20 years ago), and there was little discussion of interrelational dynamics. A more recent review by Koutra et al. (2014) repeated the focus on expressed emotion and family burden. Beyond these reviews, however, there is good evidence of the importance of taking a more systemic and relational review of family life and psychosis, and some promising indicators of where that might lead. Indeed more recent research has begun to reveal family dynamic changes from the perspective of the young person. For example, Boden-Stuart et al. (2021) examine family relationships from the perspective of the service user. Their participants described their active role in caring about/for other family members. They talked about protecting their families, whilst wishing to improve openness and communication within the family.

It has long been thought that family systems and environments have a significant impact over the course of an individuals' mental health difficulties. In the field of psychosis research, the prevailing idea has been that high levels of expressed emotion (EE) are unhelpful for recovery (Butzlaff & Hooley, 1998). High EE is characterised by a high number of critical comments, hostility or emotional over-involvement (EOI), during family interactions. Conversely, expressions of warmth and positive comments are thought to describe a 'low EE' environment. Warmth and positive remarks are frequently neglected in research (Wearden et al., 2000) and as a result, comparatively little is known about the influence of positive interactions. We do know that the impact of psychosis on relationships is one of the important consequences commonly described by service users

(McCarthy et al., 2013) and detected at follow-up in longitudinal studies (Ajnakina et al., 2021). More specifically, we can infer that one important factor contributing to this is likely to be difficulties in interpersonal communication. Such difficulties are often reported by people with psychosis (e.g. see Byrne & Morrison, 2010) and should be seen in the context of the seismic change in identity (experienced by the person with psychosis) and the narrow 'perceptual filter' which may be adopted by the family (Allman et al., 2018). To some extent, this suggests that the focus on EE (primarily parental communication) captures only one element in an important relational dynamic. In this chapter, we present analysis of family accounts of psychosis, informed by this wider, 'whole system' approach.

It is widely accepted that family interventions have an important role to play in reducing hospital admissions and relapse rates (Barrowclough & Hooley, 2003; Bird et al., 2010) and such work is widely recommended in the treatment of those diagnosed with schizophrenia (Department of Health, 2013, 2014). Currently, family therapy programmes for psychosis tend to comprise psychoeducation, problem-solving skills and crisis management (Bird et al., 2010; Pitschel-Walz et al., 2001). This may alleviate burden and help to change intrafamilial attitudes (Berglund et al., 2003), but it may also represent a missed opportunity to provide more substantive intervention and support. Unfortunately, relatively little is known about the nature of whole family relationships when one member is experiencing mental health difficulties. For example, we do not have good descriptions of familial patterns in terms of who talks to whom about what, who does what with whom, and—critically—when and how these kinds of relational activities are experienced as helpful. We do know that in the 'at risk' period prior to onset of psychosis, the dynamics of the family appear to shift, with a focus on maintaining the well-being of the young person who is experiencing distress, sometimes at the cost of other relationships and family priorities (Izon et al., 2020, 2022). Unless we understand these processes more fully, it is difficult to develop interventions which nurture the best parts of familial support.

A 'Whole Family' Study

There is a general deficit of whole family approaches, sibling and service user perspectives in existing literature regarding psychosis. This study, therefore, analysed accounts of various individuals from within the *same* family, aiming to understand roles and relationships where one member has experienced a first episode of psychosis. In particular, in this work, we wanted to understand how existing relationships and roles within families were experienced when one person has a first episode of psychosis. We were also curious to understand more about any adaptive, positive ways that families found to cope.

We decided to explore this question inductively, using Interpretative Phenomenological Analysis (IPA, Smith et al., 2009). This is an approach to qualitative inquiry chosen for its focus on the individual's interpretation of an event, privileging their own perspective and unique context (Larkin & Thompson, 2012).

Full ethical approval was awarded by the UK National Research Ethics Service. Care was taken to minimise the risk of unwanted disclosures, and identifying information was removed to ensure anonymity. We provided information about the potential for 'internal confidentiality' to be breached, and as a consequence, family members were also given the option to identify some or all of their data as 'not for quotation'.

Sixteen participants from five families were recruited, from an Early Intervention Service in the West Midlands (see Table 8.1). Family members consisted of one or both parents, the service user and in two cases, one sibling. Participants were interviewed individually where possible, to allow them to speak freely, without censoring themselves.

The length of time within the service varied from six weeks to almost three years. No families reported significant financial hardship and all lived in stable accommodation.

The sample was evenly divided by gender. Service users and siblings were aged 15–24, while the parents were 45–65+ years of age. The participating families were from white British, white other, black British and British Pakistani backgrounds.

Table 8.1 Family interviewees

Family pseudonym	Family member	Relationship
Beech	Roger	Father/Husband
	Sarah	Mother/Wife
	Annabelle	Daughter/Sister/Service user
Birch	Caroline	Mother/Wife
	John	Father/Husband
	Ben	Son/Brother
	Michael	Son/Brother/Service user
Linden	Manha	Mother/Wife
	Rafee	Son/Brother
	Safiya	Daughter/Sister/Service user
Rowan	Susan	Mother/Wife
	Martin	Father/Husband
	Jack	Son/Brother/Service user
Hawthorne	Denise	Mother/Wife
	Robert	Father/Husband
	Jo	Daughter/Sister/Service user

Data Collection and Analysis

An interview topic guide, designed by the researchers in collaboration with a carer who was not involved with the research, was used to prompt discussion. The explicit aim was to discuss the nature of family relationships and what, if any, changes had occurred since the onset of psychosis. Questions were open-ended and often circular (e.g. "How do other members of the family feel about that?"), designed to encourage exploration of the family.

Interview transcripts were interrogated using IPA as described in Smith et al. (2009). An iterative process of collating and grouping individual and family level themes was completed, convergence or divergence and isolated constructs were observed and superordinate themes developed. We attempted to identify and manage our own assumptions, given best practice of reflexivity (Ahern, 1999). We do, however, acknowledge our implicit presumptions that families are important and mutually influential.

From the interviews, we identified and developed three main themes: "Adapting through learning and communicating", "Unity, sharing and delegating" and "Damage, repair and revisiting". These describe how families adapted to the changes that resulted from the psychosis through learning and communication, and how dynamics between individuals affected the family system, and thus operated to sustain the family as a unit.

Adapting Through Learning and Communicating: From 'Not Talking' to 'Trying to Understand'

This theme describes how, in the process of learning of their loved one's difficulties, coming to understand them and how to support them, individuals tended to take different roles. Some family members actively researched the issue, and others preferred to take a more passive approach.

The extremely unfamiliar nature of the condition was difficult to understand and so most family members had a desire to better understand what their relative was experiencing. They found that learning increases understanding, and they described benefitting from educating themselves. They did this by attending classes, by researching online, by talking to mental health professionals, and from personal reflection. For example, mother Susan Rowan described how *"I thought 'I'd like to see what it's like'. … I've sat there and tried to hear voices, I'll try anything!"*. Another benefit came from developing empathy and reducing frustration, as husband and father Martin Rowan explained while talking about improving his understanding of psychotic illness through attending a carers' group:

> *It also makes us understand what Jack's going through a bit more. […] So that, that's been quite a big help to us I think. […] It makes you more tolerant I think to the situation rather than kind of, to start with you're almost, I'd be banging my head against the wall almost, in … in … in the sense that I couldn't get my head around why he was doing it.*

In this way, information and family therapy from EI services were frequently described as being helpful.

Others took a less active approach. For example, Robert Hawthorn, father of Jo, actively avoided informative materials, preferring to take a 'wait and see' approach, in contrast to the more interrogative style of others in the family unit:

> *I say, "Look, don't put too much into your mind because erm you can self-diagnosis wrong too much," you know. And I'm not convinced yet that it is anything to do with psychosis.*

This contrasting approach potentially allows the family to maintain some balance or sense of normality through a kind of 'naive optimism' about the situation. It may moderate the emotional tone, but only if it is not in conflict with other family members' views, or unfolding events.

Across the interviews, however, there was a general sense that families appreciated the value of learning, because it was perceived to facilitate understanding and empathy. They ascribed the benefits of communication/sharing to what they had learned. Families recognised that poor communication did not benefit anyone, as difficulties remained unspoken, leaving problems to grow, causing relational strain. As sibling Ben Birch described:

> *It used to be we'd just keep it to ourself and stuff, and like, that'd mean the problems would get worse. We'd be in a mood and be like, "Oh what's wrong?" "Nothing, nothing is wrong" and then, but really something was wrong, but we wouldn't be talking.*

Clear and frequent communication was valued because it brought closeness, a sense of unity and a more supportive atmosphere. It also enabled relatives to work together towards resolutions, as Ben continued:

> *The ups are also that he can vent it because that means that he's not keeping it to himself, he sort of… we're, like, we can help each other feel better by talking to each other.*

Unity, Sharing and Delegating: Facing Difficulty Together

This superordinate theme encapsulates the feeling of the family being a unit, functioning with a shared goal in mind and delegating tasks according to ability. Some participants spoke of this as something that was limited to the nuclear family, but two families were sufficiently close with extended family to include them in their idea of the family as a unit. As such, the well-being of the group was seen as dependent upon the well-being of individuals, as John Birch explained: *"These things wax and wane. Any, any sort of dip affects us all"*. Therefore, the impact of the FEP rippled throughout the unit, meaning the needs of all had to be addressed, as he continued: "*Mental health is four times more expensive in this house because there's four people to look after rather than just one*".

While the episode was depicted as difficult, families described how relationships had been strained but grown stronger. Perhaps that shared impact and shared purpose of recovery united the family further and contributed towards the development of even closer relationships, as Martin Rowan described: *"Everyone's been drawn into the fact that we have to kind of look after each other, we have to look after Jack. So in some senses I think it'll probably make us stronger"*. This was an idea also reflected by his wife, and shared amongst other families. Furthermore, experiencing difficulty together appeared to provide depth and shared understandings:

> *Obviously we've been facing it together and discussing it and, and praying about it and all that, and so I think, yes it's, it, it's been much the same, perhaps strengthening and deepenings as well.*

Here Roger Beech (father and husband) seems to outline how good relationships have been reaffirmed through shared experience, where mutual support and open communication are a key feature. This is closely linked with seeing the family as a unit where the well-being of the group is dependent upon the well-being of all individuals. Families shared and delegated roles such as 'organiser' or 'confidant', which were flexibly assumed according to suitability:

> *I'm no expert but I'm quite happy to be considered the expert because it helps people have a central point to talk to, whether I am is [laughs] you know, debatable.* (John Birch)

Here this family, in common with some others, organised itself around the allocation of a role that provides a framework for discussing specific issues.

Especially close relationship pairings frequently emerged as being helpful within the family. These special connections and secret languages revealed ways of being with one another where secrets could be shared and a close bond fostered. In the example below, Michael Birch, son, sibling and service user, describes reciprocal behaviours to enjoy shared pleasures that create a unique, secret bond between himself and his brother:

> *We always do things like that [getting each other little presents] and I like that, it's nice and we get each other like little presents and like that, we'll do that with my parents but [whispers] they don't always like us eating sweets and stuff so… it's kind of a little, secret brotherly thing that they don't know about [laughs].*

This bond is distinct within the family and was recognised by others in the family as a special relationship. It was a common theme among the families that special bonds developed through sharing interests and private things. Facilitating factors included similarities in age or gender, simply being available and spending time together in a relaxed way, contributing towards a shared understanding: *"we just, we get each other and it's good"* (Michael Birch). Often these connections were enacted and maintained through specific relational attributes (being open, for example) or through particular relational behaviours (helping, giving advice, for example).

An important mechanism for some relationships was the 'shared interest'. Mother Sarah Beech described an important example from her family:

> *Sport is their language so they'll have those conversations and, […] as [son] has got older they've grown closer and in that way, finding sort of [laughs] finding a language. […][son] is much more of an introvert, more like me but, so perhaps that's why I notice the sporting language that they share [laughs].*

Here, sport provides a platform upon which a parent and child can spend time together. In this way, most family members shared a unique connection with each other that was reasonably exclusive and facilitated time together. Spending time with one another was a cornerstone from which close relationships were built. Through this, families were at least able to support each other by being close and providing normality, independent of the ups and downs of psychosis.

Ultimately the families considered themselves to be a cohesive unit. Shared goals appeared to be organised within the group. Their special languages seemed to facilitate relationships and through this, provided relief from more demanding relationships: e.g. *"we have all tried to fix things that others have felt could be inconvenient or cause disruption and … negativity"* (son, Michael Birch). These opportunities for relief and repair enabled individuals to perform reciprocal helping roles and create bonding experiences, whilst feeling sufficiently relaxed to be themselves without pressure, and being accepted as such.

Damage, Repair and Revisit: Maintaining Balance in the Family System

Perhaps as a result of stress brought on by the episode, conflict or difficult relationships sometimes emerged. However, where there was damage to relationships, this was noticed by the family system, and efforts to repair were made in various ways. For example, other members of the family more passively provided light-hearted relief or took active roles in counterbalancing or repairing fractious interactions as John Birch noted:

> *We could almost be a good cop bad cop setup, […] often if Caroline's having a rant or a moan about something with Michael or Ben, I tend to let them take the other op, the other point of view, not to be contrary to Caroline but to try*

and "look you know, actually, this is, this is tough love and I'm just trying to show the love bit".

Furthermore, John's son, Michael who had experienced a FEP, revealed that he noticed this action. In this way, efforts were made to relieve the directly involved individuals of stress and alleviate a negative environment. Some took the role of protecting the service user by defending their behaviours and helping others to understand their difficulties.

As the episode revealed an increased vulnerability in the individual, relatives responded with more active or intensive parenting as required. Participants described their loved one becoming more dependent upon them, causing them to revisit stages of development that were reminiscent of earlier childhood: *"we first went to the doctors when he was 14 and he sat on my husband's knee and I read out all the things that Jack was doing and he became like a little baby again, you know".* Here, Susan Rowan describes vulnerability in her son, illustrating the increased reliance on his parents. For some families, this felt like a natural behaviour, but for others, it could be frustrating or uncomfortable and difficult to manage appropriately, for example:

We don't wanna keep going "Are you ok?" because then he, he'll say, "Oh don't patronise me" or whatever. So, we have to be careful. (Ben Birch, sibling)

Even younger siblings can be recruited into a responsible caring role, and it can be difficult to strike the right balance between caring, and being perceived as over-involved or annoying. How this was experienced by the service user depended upon the understanding of their needs and their relatives' intentions. While Ben highlights how caring could be annoying, several service users described it as reassuring and helpful. Indeed, a son sitting on his father's knee, as Susan Rowan described, is an active attempt to elicit such care. Those who did experience increased parenting as annoying acknowledged in hindsight that this had been appropriate and even necessary. Susan's son Jack, who experienced psychosis, reflected: *"it [parental caretaking] needs to be done".* There seems to be a complex quality to this interaction. We might think of it as something to be worked through like partners in a dance, where the relative needs to be sensitive to the wants and needs of the service user, and also able to meet those needs in ways that respect their developmental stage.

This theme encapsulates how the family system can balance or maintain individual relationships within the family and simultaneously progress toward family goals as a whole. Where strain begins to cause damage, functional roles (such as organiser, resident expert, etc.) can relieve stress and help bring order to chaos and sense making to confusion. Attachment type roles (such as caregiver, confidant, etc.) may be revisited and may help to create safety and containment in frightening circumstances. Thus, these micro dynamics support actors/players within the system, and this consequently supports the health of the system as a whole.

Reflections

The aim of this study was to gain insights into family systems during a FEP. The superordinate themes describe how the family system reacts, adapts and finds a way of moving forward with the disruption that FEP can bring. Families' intensity of support also varied substantially in relation to their loved one's stage of recovery.

Family Resilience

Although the episode was very difficult, nevertheless some families described having been drawn closer together and become more unified as a result. Facing challenges together and experiencing positive adaptation and growth are perhaps ways of describing a resilient response within the family's experience of mental health difficulties (Marsh et al., 1996). Indeed, resilience may best be understood as a property of systems rather than individuals. It has been described as "The successful coping of families during life transitions, stress, or adversity" (Black & Lobo, 2008, p. 33) and has been identified as a possible factor in the family's experience of mental health difficulties (Marsh et al., 1996). One way of reading our study is that it provides a snapshot of what familial resilience looks like—having the adaptive capacity to regroup and reconfigure in response to a problem, and providing additional support to an individual in the system when they need it, through sharing and delegating, and repairing and revisiting. These responses share many of the characteristics of resilient families described by Black and Lobo (2008) such as family member accord (coherence, nurturance), flexibility and communication. The idea that families felt that they had grown in some way, through their response, suggests that there may be a useful analogy to be drawn with the growth that can occur at an individual level after traumatic stress (Joseph & Linley, 2006).

It is important to note that the families in this study were 'intact', and supporting a family member who had been in distress for a relatively short time. The capacity of a system to demonstrate resilience over time is likely to be reduced by attrition, unless there is respite and replenishment. Thus, our study did not investigate the entire range of possible experiences of families experiencing FEP, particularly more fragmented or ruptured systems, but it does offer a useful perspective on what 'good' can look like.

Connections

An important feature of this effective and adaptive regrouping is concerned with how families maintained their connections and demonstrated care. The 'special connections' which participants identified showed how highly valued some small, thoughtful gestures can be. The association between silent connections and affective communication in close relationships has been previously discussed by Gabb et al. (2013), in the context of romantic relationships. The sense of being special for someone and held in mind by them is important because we know that loneliness is a major problem for people with psychosis (Lim et al., 2018). Interventions targeting social isolation have demonstrated good clinical outcomes (Saunders, 2003). We would therefore encourage clinical services to promote interventions designed to support the fostering of such relationships.

Social support is important to individual and family resilience (Black & Lobo, 2008; Southwick et al., 2005), and resilience has been proposed to enable the individual to protect themselves from criticism or over-involvement (Miklowitz, 2004), so perhaps these special relationships help counterbalance, or alleviate, more difficult relationships. Some of the factors (such as availability, reciprocity, etc.) underpinning these special relationships are reminiscent of core values in secure attachment patterns (Ainsworth et al., 1978; Danquah & Berry, 2014). The active behaviours described in the themes (e.g. repair, revisit, care-seeking, responding) all reflect qualities described as essential in secure attachments (Ainsworth et al., 1978; Marvin et al., 2002).

The attachment system is stimulated by threatening events such as illness (Bowlby, 1969; Gumley et al., 2014). In the context of literature which has previously questioned the inappropriateness of emotional 'over-involvement', we might suggest that where more intensive care is elicited, it is in fact appropriate. However, this does require a fine balance on behalf of the caregiver to demonstrate qualities such as availability and sensitive responsiveness in order to recognise care-seeking and exploration-seeking behaviours (Ainsworth et al., 1978). Perhaps it is where care is not sensitively responsive that a mismatch between desired and received level of care occurs and difficulties arise. This study therefore highlights the value of an attachment-oriented approach in guiding clinicians and family members' interactions with service users.

While the experience of the onset of a FEP was widely regarded as an extremely difficult time, families in our study made active attempts to understand and make sense of it. While they experienced significant strain, they also made efforts to repair interpersonal difficulties, while sharing responsibilities and working together towards a common goal which brought them closer. Further exploration of how family systems operate and respond during FEP and recovery should be a priority for psychosis research. There are promising indicators here of what a resilient response might look like, but this needs to be augmented by a developmental picture (e.g. how does the response change over time, and under duress?) and in the contexts of different familial structures and living arrangements. It is also important—of course—to be able to describe the common things which can go wrong when families are coping with psychosis. The implications of a more fully developed view of these dynamics should be instrumental to intervention development and service improvement. In many psychosis services, behavioural family therapy is already a means of providing some psychoeducation and family support. This intervention can be an effective component of multi-disciplinary responses (when it is delivered), but it speaks more directly to addressing some of the issues around communication *deficits* than it does to building the *strengths* described by the families in our study (e.g. unity, balance, special relationships). There is the potential to work with families to co-design new interventions which—for example—draw on attachment theories to help families to maintain balance (e,g. in meeting the needs of all young people in the family), or which draw on team-building approaches to help them to develop shared purpose and unity (e.g. when under stress and strain).

Acknowledgements The first author would like to express her gratitude to the families who agreed to participate in this research during some of the most challenging times in their lives, and also to give thanks to her co-authors for their support.

References

Ahern, K. J. (1999). Ten tips for reflexive bracketing. *Qualitative Health Research, 9*(3), 407–411. https://doi.org/10.1177/104973299129121947

Ainsworth, M. D. S., Blehar, M. C., Waters, E., & Wall, S. (1978). *Patterns of attachment: A psychological study of the strange situation*. Lawrence Erlbaum Associates.

Ajnakina, O., Stubbs, B., Francis, E., Gaughran, F., David, A. S., Murray, R. M., & Lally, J. (2021). Employment and relationship outcomes in first-episode psychosis: A systematic review and meta-analysis of longitudinal studies. *Schizophrenia Research, 231*, 122–133.

Allman, J. J. P., Cooke, A., Whitfield, B., & McCartney, M. (2018). "It doesn't mean I'm useless" how do young people experiencing psychosis contribute to their families and why are their contributions sometimes overlooked? *Psychosis: Psychological Social and Integrative Approaches, 10*, 11–21.

Amaresha, A. C., & Venkatasubramanian, G. (2012). Expressed emotion in schizophrenia: An overview. *Indian Journal of Psychological Medicine, 34*(1), 12–20. https://doi.org/10.4103/0253

Barrowclough, C., & Hooley, J. M. (2003). Attributions and expressed emotion: A review. *Clinical Psychology Review, 23*(6), 849–880. https://doi.org/10.1016/S0272-7358(03)00075-8

Berglund, N., Vahlne, J. O., & Edman, A. (2003). Family intervention in schizophrenia—Impact on family burden and attitude. *Social Psychiatry and Psychiatric Epidemiology, 38*(3), 116–121. https://doi.org/10.1007/s00127-003-0615-6

Bird, V., Premkumar, P., Kendall, T., Whittington, C., Mitchell, J., & Kuipers, E. (2010). Early intervention services, cognitive-behavioural therapy and family intervention in early psychosis: Systematic review. *The British Journal of Psychiatry: The Journal of Mental Science, 197*(5), 350–356. https://doi.org/10.1192/bjp.bp.109.074526

Black, K., & Lobo, M. (2008). Family resilience factors. *Journal of Family Nursing, 14*(1), 33–55. https://doi.org/10.1177/1074840707312237

Boden-Stuart, Z. V. R., Larkin, M., & Harrop, C. (2021). Young adults' dynamic relationships with their families in early psychosis: Identifying relational strengths and supporting relational agency. *Psychology and Psychotherapy: Theory, Research and Practice, 94*, 646–666. https://doi.org/10.1111/papt.12337

Bowlby, J. (1969). *Attachment and loss, volume 1: Attachment*. Pimlico.

Butzlaff, R. L., & Hooley, J. M. (1998). Expressed emotion and psychiatric relapse: A meta-analysis. *Archives of General Psychiatry, 55*(6), 547–552. https://doi.org/10.1001/archpsyc.55.6.547

Byrne, R., & Morrison, A. P. (2010). Young people at risk of psychosis: A user-led exploration of interpersonal relationships and communication of psychological difficulties. *Early Intervention in Psychiatry, 4*, 162–168. https://doi.org/10.1111/j.1751-7893.2010.00171.xB

Danquah, A. N., & Berry, K. (2014). *Attachment theory in adult mental health: A guide to clinical practice*. Routledge.

Department of Health. (2013). *Psychosis and schizophrenia in children and young people: Recognition and management.*

Department of Health. (2014). Psychosis and schizophrenia in adults: Treatment and management. .

Gabb, J., Klett-Davies, M., Fink, J., & Thomae, M. (2013). *Enduring love? Couple relationships in the 21st century.* Retrieved from http://www.open.ac.uk/researchprojects/enduringlove/files/enduringlove/file/ecms/web-content/Final-Enduring-Love-Survey-Report.pdf

Gumley, A. I., Taylor, H. E. F., Schwannauer, M., & MacBeth, A. (2014). A systematic review of attachment and psychosis: Measurement, construct validity and outcomes. *Acta Psychiatrica Scandinavica, 129*(4), 257–274. https://doi.org/10.1111/acps.12172

Harrop, C., & Trower, P. (2001). Why does schizophrenia develop at late adolescence? *Clinical Psychology Review, 21*(2), 241–265. https://doi.org/10.1016/S0272-7358(99)00047-1

Izon, E., Berry, K., Law, H., Shiers, D., & French, P. (2020). "I don't think I took her fears seriously": Exploring the experiences of family members of individuals at-risk of developing psychosis over 12 months. *Clinical Psychology & Psychotherapy, 27*, 965–976. https://doi.org/10.1002/cpp.2483

Izon, E., Berry, K., Law, H., & French, P. (2022). 'If he feels better I'll feel better' relationships with individuals at high-risk of developing psychosis. *Early Intervention in Psychiatry, 16*, 231–238. https://doi.org/10.1111/eip.13146

Joseph, S., & Linley, P. A. (2006). Growth following adversity: Theoretical perspectives and implications for clinical practice. *Clinical Psychology Review, 26*(8), 1041–1053.

Jungbauer, J., Stelling, K., Dietrich, S., & Angermeyer, M. C. (2004). Schizophrenia: Problems of separation in families. *Journal of Advanced Nursing, 47*(6), 605–613. https://doi.org/10.1111/j.1365-2648.2004.03157.x

Koutra, K., Vgontzas, A. N., Lionis, C., et al. (2014). Family functioning in first-episode psychosis: a systematic review of the literature. *Social Psychiatry and Psychiatric Epidemiology, 49*, 1023–1036. https://doi.org/10.1007/s00127-013-0816-6

Larkin, M., & Thompson, A. R. (2012). Interpretative phenomenological analysis in mental health and psychotherapy research. In *Qualitative research methods in mental health and psychotherapy: A guide for students and practitioners* (pp. 99–116).

Lim, M. H., Gleeson, J. F. M., Alvarez-Jimenez, M., et al. (2018). Loneliness in psychosis: a systematic review. *Social Psychiatry and Psychiatric Epidemiology, 53*, 221–238. https://doi.org/10.1007/s00127-018-1482-5

Marsh, D. T., Lefley, H. P., EvansRhodes, D., Ansell, V. I., Doerzbacher, B. M., LaBarbera, L., & Paluzzi, J. E. (1996). The family experience of mental illness: Evidence for resilience. *Psychiatric Rehabilitation Journal, 20*(2), 3–12. Retrieved from //a1996wd18800002.

Marvin, R., Cooper, G., Hoffman, K., & Powell, B. (2002). The Circle of Security project: Attachment-based intervention with caregiver-pre-school child dyads. *Attachment & Human Development, 4*(1), 107–124. https://doi.org/10.1080/14616730252982491

McCarthy-Jones, S., Marriott, M., Knowles, R., Rowse, G., & Thompson, A. R. (2013). What is psychosis? A meta-synthesis of inductive qualitative studies exploring the experience of psychosis. *Psychosis, 5*(1), 1–16. https://doi.org/10.1080/17522439.2011.647051

Miklowitz, D. J. (2004). The role of family systems in severe and recurrent psychiatric disorders: A developmental psychopathology view. *Development and Psychopathology, 16*(3), 667–88. Retrieved from http://www.ncbi.nlm.nih.gov/pubmed/15605631

Pitschel-Walz, G., Leucht, S., Bäuml, J., Kissling, W., & Engel, R. R. (2001). The effect of family interventions on relapse and rehospitalization in schizophrenia—A meta-analysis. *Schizophrenia Bulletin, 27*(1), 73–92. Retrieved from https://frodon.univ-paris5.fr/url?, http://search.ebscohost.com/login.aspx?direct=true&db=pdh&AN=2001-16630-007&lang=fr&site=ehost-live/, http://content.ebscohost.com/ContentServer.asp?T=P&P=AN&K=2001-16630-007&S=L&D=pdh&EbscoContent=dGJyMMvl7ESeprA4y9fwOLCm

Saunders, J. C. (2003). Families living with severe mental illness: A literature review. *Issues in Mental Health Nursing, 24*(2), 175–198. https://doi.org/10.1080/01612840390160711

Smith, J. A., Flowers, P., & Larkin, M. (2009). *Interpretative phenomenological analysis: Theory, method and research*. Sage.

Southwick, S. M., Vythilingam, M., & Charney, D. S. (2005). The psychobiology of depression and resilience to stress: Implications for prevention and treatment. *Annual Review of Clinical Psychology, 1*, 255–291. https://doi.org/10.1146/annurev.clinpsy.1.102803.143948

Wearden, A. J., Tarrier, N., Barrowclough, C., Zastowny, T. R., & Rahill, A. A. (2000). A review of expressed emotion research in health care. *Clinical Psychology Review, 20*(5), 633–666. https://doi.org/10.1016/S0272-7358(99)00008-2

9

Relatedness and Connectedness Over Time: How Young People Make Sense of Their Relationships During Their Recovery from First-Episode Psychosis

Amy Symonds, Mark Bernard, Andrew Fox, and Michael Larkin

'Psychosis' refers to a range of experiences, thought to lie on a continuum, which often include hearing voices or sensing things that others do not, holding strong beliefs that are not commonly shared, having difficulties with thinking and concentrating, and difficulties with motivation (Cooke, 2017). The British Psychological Society (2017) estimates that around a million people in the United Kingdom have a psychiatric

A. Symonds (✉)
Worcestershire Acute Hospitals NHS Trust, Worcester, UK
e-mail: a.symonds3@nhs.net

M. Bernard
Birmingham Early Intervention in Psychosis Service, Birmingham, UK

A. Fox
University of Birmingham, Birmingham, UK

M. Larkin
Aston University, Birmingham, UK

Z. Boden-Stuart, M. Larkin (eds.), *Relationships and Mental Health*,
https://doi.org/10.1007/978-3-031-50047-3_9

diagnosis which is likely to include such experiences. Psychosis is often distressing and debilitating, and people experiencing psychosis have a higher-than-average risk of self-harm and suicide (NHS, 2019).

The Developmental and Relational Context of First-Episode Psychosis

Young people aged between 14 and 35 are suggested to be most at risk of developing psychosis, with a median age of 22 years at first onset (Cheng et al., 2011). Often coinciding with the formative developmental stage of 'Emerging Adulthood' (Arnett, 2000), psychosis poses distinct challenges for young people (Windell & Norman, 2012), and the first 3–5 years following onset are thought to represent a 'critical period' for determining longer-term outcomes (Crumlish et al., 2009; Linszen & Birchwood, 2000).

At the typical age of onset for a first episode of psychosis (FEP), young people are often exploring new relationships and social roles with peers and partners (e.g. Bagwell et al., 2005), an important stage linked with the development of a sense of relatedness to others (e.g. Blatt & Luyten, 2009) and with consolidating personal identity (e.g. Erikson, 1963; Arnett, 2000). Whilst emerging adulthood is associated with increasing autonomy and individuation (Harrop & Trower, 2003), healthy development is also thought to be facilitated by maintaining emotional connectedness with parents (Moretti & Peled, 2004). This 'parallel development' of autonomy and relatedness, which leads to the integration and consolidation of self and relationships, is central for wellbeing (Arnett, 2000).

The NICE guidelines (2014) recognise that psychosis can impact not only upon the individual but also upon family and friends, and that the experience of psychosis can be linked with a decline in social functioning, a reduced social network, and fewer friends (Macdonald et al., 2000). This is particularly significant given the developmental context of FEP, in addition to the human drive to form significant and lasting relationships (Baumeister & Leary, 1995). NICE (2014) recognises that others are important in the long-term recovery process, and the Quality Standards for Early Intervention in Psychosis Services (Baugh & Lucas-Motley, 2021) suggest that young people should be supported to develop their social networks by services that promote social inclusion and tackle isolation.

Relatedness, Connectedness, and Recovery from First-Episode Psychosis

Although increased independence is often sought during young adulthood, the need for connectedness does not lessen. Woodman and McArthur suggest instead that it 'evolves' (2017), with young people's relational needs and expectations maturing and changing during this period. Perhaps surprisingly, feelings of loneliness are now thought to peak in adolescence (Mann et al., 2017), with lonelier young people more likely to experience mental health problems, and to attempt suicide (Matthews et al., 2018). Loneliness is highlighted in ultra-high-risk-for-psychosis states, whilst 80% of people with a diagnosis of psychosis report loneliness as a 'major challenge' (Mann et al., 2017), with over a third identifying loneliness as a barrier to recovery (Lim & Gleeson, 2014). Loneliness is both an experience of absence (meaningful connections with others are missing; Motta & Larkin, 2022) and of presence (of the sense that these connections are available for other people; Kidd, 2022). The high prevalence of loneliness amongst young adults underscores the importance of relationality to their wellbeing.

A review of the conceptualisation of personal recovery has emphasised the importance of connectedness to others (Leamy et al., 2011), which is thought to be 'vital' to recovery (Tew et al., 2012). A strong association has been found between social connection and mental health in adolescence, with social networks adding significant explanatory power to outcomes (Levula et al., 2016). Following FEP, relationships which provide a sense of relatedness and value, as enacted by a variety of sources, have been found to be the most frequently cited positive influence upon recovery, enhancing wellbeing in a variety of ways (Windell & Norman, 2012).

Support from friends in particular is suggested to be an important positive predictor of both immediate and longer-term resilience in young people (van Harmelen et al., 2017), whilst poor friendships may be a causal and maintenance factor for psychotic symptoms (Harrop et al., 2014). It is not surprising, then, that people seek out positive relationships and social environments as a way of managing their symptoms, therefore aiding recovery (Schön et al., 2009).

Through discussion of interview data with young people, this chapter will consider how young people make meaning of their relationships with others in relation to their recovery from FEP, and how such relationships may influence the recovery process. We will explore temporal aspects of relationships, from a more 'acute' phase of psychosis to the recovery phase, and how young people's relationships may be understood and utilised differently over time.

Relatedness and Connectedness Over Time

The first author conducted in-depth, semi-structured interviews with eight young people in the emerging adulthood stage of development, who had experienced FEP within the last five years. Some of the young people felt they had recovered, while others expressed being in the process of recovery. All of the young people touched upon co-existing mental health difficulties, which is consistent with the high rates of emotional difficulties documented in FEP samples (Birchwood, 2003). The young people were continuing to receive care and support from an inner-city Early Intervention for Psychosis service. The sample was ethnically and culturally diverse, and they were aged between 18 and 23. Ethical approval was granted after review by the National Research Ethics Service (NRES). Names used here in the text are all pseudonyms created by the first author. Names used in images are all pseudonyms created by the participant.

We invited the young people to take part in two interviews: the first was retrospective, inviting conversation about the experience of psychosis and relationships during the time the young people felt most unwell. The second interview invited conversation about current experiences of recovery and relationships. Meeting the young people on two occasions appeared to deepen rapport with and trust in the first author, which in turn supported the young people in providing rich descriptions of their experiences.

All interview transcripts were analysed utilising an Interpretative Phenomenological Analysis (IPA) approach according to Smith's (2012) guidelines. This is a qualitative research approach that is "committed to the examination of how people make sense of their major life experiences" (Smith et al., 2012, p. 1), with a specific focus on the perception of experience. The IPA researcher attempts to make sense of the participant making sense of their experiences and the world around them, thus engaging in a double hermeneutic. Examining the meanings which individuals attach to their experience "may illuminate the embodied, cognitive-affective and existential domains" of a person's lifeworld (Smith et al., 2012, p. 34), and thus IPA was felt to be an appropriate and suitable approach, enabling a rich exploration of how young people make sense of their relationships in the context of their recovery from FEP.

Visual methods were incorporated within the interviews. We provided the young people with paper and coloured pens, and invited them to create a visual representation of their relational networks. Boden et al. (2018) note that visual methodologies are consonant with IPA principles, and that relational experience in particular lends itself well to visual representation, allowing "the 'unspeakable' to reveal itself" (Kirova & Emme, 2006, p. 4). Creation of the maps appeared to support engagement, offering an additional 'way in' to reflect upon experience which was "non-linguistic, and directly intertwined with the felt-sense" (Boden & Eatough, 2014, p. 163). The visual representations of the young peoples' relational networks were analysed individually, in pairs (across interviews), and as an overall set (across participants), enabling the identification of commonalities and differences. Certain questions were considered for each representation, based on the analysis framework suggested by Boden et al. (2018).

In the remainder of the chapter, we discuss six themes which we developed from the young people's accounts:

1. Relationships Can Thrive or Wither
2. Re-constructing the Self in Relation to Others

3. Shifting Between Dependence and Independence
4. Relationship Re-appraisal and Re-evaluation
5. The Evolution of Others' Sense-Making
6. Re-engaging with a Reciprocal Network

Relationships Can Thrive or Wither

Many of the young people reflected upon the thriving or withering of their relationships, following the onset of psychosis and during their recovery process. The strengthening of bonds and increased closeness is often facilitated by a sense of increased emotional intimacy, following others having experienced "the inside out of everything" as articulated by Radhiya:

> *[I'm now closer to] my mum … definitely my mum […] she's been through the whole experience with me, she's seen the inside out of everything, through night and day […] she used to stay up with me, late in the night until I'd fall asleep … and, she's just went through everything positive with me, like, through the whole thing … she encouraged me to get out of this whole isolation thing that I went through.*

Radhiya additionally highlights that recovery from psychosis provides opportunities to share positive experiences, such as a shared sense of achievement, which appears to also strengthen relational bonds. Ellie extends this further, reflecting that sharing in a very profound experience (psychosis and a suicide attempt) appears to have increased both her and her friend's 'knowing' of each other. Ellie's emotional expression highlights the gratitude she feels for her friend and their relationship:

> *When I took the overdose, [my friend] was the one who took me to hospital, so … that made us even closer, our friendship, after that … so … she's been absolutely key as well. … I mean she saved my life in that instance, probably … 'cause they said that my heart stopped beating so … maybe if I hadn't have gone to hospital when I did … so … I'm really emotional again [becomes tearful]*

[…] she knows so much about me, like so much, she's been there through a lot of the things I've been through.

In contrast to the preceding accounts, the young people also talked about the withering of relationships. For Achara, friendships from university had weakened, following a period of social isolation, whilst for Jamie, relationships with family members had become strained in the context of differing expectations and appraisals of Jamie's recovery progress. For Sana, we can see how her perception that male family members were not there for her when she needed them has resulted in a sense of emotional withdrawal and disconnection, leaving a 'hole' in Sana's life and a sense of loss of her relationships with her father and brothers:

They ask all these intrusive questions, as if they have a right, like just because they're my brothers, or my dad or whatever, like, they were never there when I needed them, and now […] that I'm relatively okay, well, in their eyes, um … they kinda abuse their authority over me, I don't know, it's weird 'cause, […] I can't explain it, because, in a sense it doesn't impact in my everyday life, and um, because I don't think about it, and I don't think about them, because I don't like thinking about them, but then it does kind of impact it because I don't really have any brother figures or a father figure or anything.

Re-constructing the Self in Relation to Others

During analysis, the relational context within which the young people make sense of their experiences and themselves became evident. In turn, this often involves a process of re-constructing the sense of self. How others related and responded to the young people during their experience of psychosis and recovery had a profound effect upon how they understood themselves:

Jamie: I had loads of relationships, I had loads of friends, some closer than the other. […] I couldn't walk anywhere without seeing someone I know … and like they'd have time for me, you know if you're seeing them and you're like in a sort of position or situation where you can stop, they'd have the time for me and they'd stop and they'd chat and like, I just found that like, after, like, what freaked me out is like people just didn't have the time for me and whether it was because, like, they thought, you know, I was a bit fragile from what had happened and stuff but you know, like, even like close mates, you know, like … like people that I'd done a lot of things with, had a lot of experiences with, like, they just, ain't got the time of day for me … and like, that, that's what messes with your head, 'cause you think, like, what have I done?

Here Jamie describes changes in how others related to him following the onset of psychosis, which felt confusing and unsettling, highlighting an incongruence between the way others saw him and how he saw himself. Challenges to perceived social acceptance are greatest after a *first* episode of psychosis (Birchwood, 2003), when young people tend to be more ego-centric (Harrop & Trower, 2003). In Jamie's case, these challenges led him to question his fragility and, ultimately, to wonder whether he was to blame. The young people understanding themselves through the eyes of others aligns with Cooley's concept of the 'looking glass self' (1967) and theory of the self as essentially social, whereby people imagine what they look like to others, before incorporating what they imagine into their self-concept. Cooley described how 'self-feelings' arise from this process (e.g. pride or shame). Such feelings were discussed by many of the young people in our study and framed as either supporting *or* hindering their recovery. What seems especially important here is the *potential* for others to reflect a self which is sufficient and secure.

More commonly, the young people discussed the other side of this. Like Jamie, Ellie experienced someone else's view of her as vulnerable:

My mum's reactions to things, which she can't help, and her feelings are valid, but like over the summer I told her I was hearing voices again and she was crying, not in front of me, but crying later, and it made me so angry, which is not fair on her, but […] it doesn't have to be something to get so upset about, when you get so upset it makes me feel like I'm ill, or there's something wrong with me again, […] actually you know I'm dealing with it, maybe not perfectly but it's not the end of the world, but sometimes the reaction does make it feel like it's the end of the world […] maybe if someone helped her see that it's really not the end of the world … or … even if I never get 'better' in the traditional sense, it's not … you know it's not the end of the world. … I think that would be nice. … I think that, that would help … and … yeah, treating, making me feel like I'm ill sometimes just doesn't help … but you know there's a balance between accepting that you are so that you can get help.

Ellie is trying to make sense of her mum making sense of the re-emergence of voice-hearing. Ellie conveys a sense of acceptance whilst feeling that her mum had experienced the same situation as something more devastating: "the end of the world". Ellie spoke passionately about this, expressing how her mum's response had led her to feel that there was "something wrong with me". There is an attempt to balance an acceptance of her difficulties in order to engage with support, with not wanting to be defined by an 'illness', which was referred to by many of the young people. Understanding and addressing mental health stigma remains important, as felt stigma can discourage help-seeking (Griffiths et al., 2019; Thornicroft et al., 2007) and influence disengagement from services during transition from Early Intervention to Adult Mental Health services (McNamara et al., 2017).

For others, re-constructing the sense of self in relation to others carries more hopeful tones. At Time 1, Sana drew a striking image of her auntie and mum either side of her, implying a sense of unity and solidarity, with shading highlighting relational meaning. At Time 2, Sana included quotes representing key messages instilled by her auntie and mum, which carry tones of love, acceptance, and empowerment, and which appear to have been internalised during Sana's recovery process (Fig. 9.1).

The family tree-like structure at Time 2 suggests a hierarchy, with Sana taking top position, giving the impression of a robust sense of self *and* connectedness. However, unlike at Time 1, Sana's school friends and hospital friends are not included at Time 2, representing a withering of these networks over time:

The people I was in hospital with […] now, they're all at college or university or […] something like that, […] they're doing something with their lives, and it kind of makes me feel bad, and that's why I've stopped talking to the majority of them, like I had loads of their numbers. […] I love seeing my friends get better, […] I really do, […] it makes me happy, but, it also makes me think about myself, like, what I could have achieved and what I didn't achieve … and it kinda makes me feel bad.

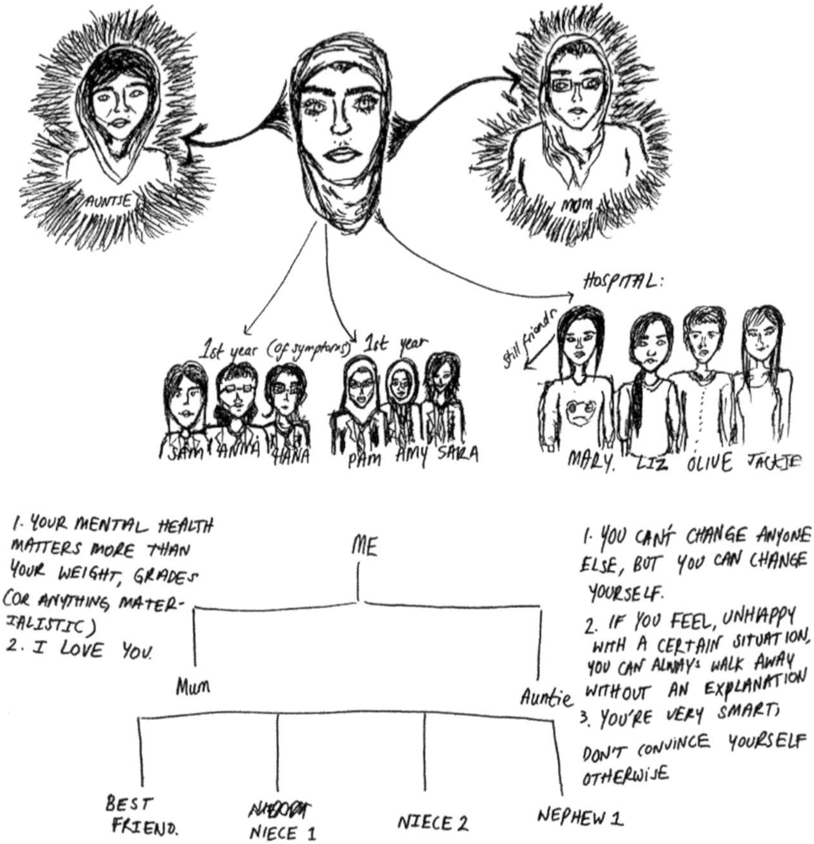

Fig. 9.1 Sana's image at Time 2

We can see that, just as the young people see themselves through the eyes of others, how the young people feel about themselves also influences how they then connect with others. Sana describes becoming aware of the 'progress' of other young people, which shone a light upon her own perceived lack of progress in comparison to them. This is in keeping with 'social rank' theory (Gilbert, 2002) which suggests that our perceived place in the world, in relation to others, is important for wellbeing. Sana also spoke about feeling lonely: social rank theory would invite us to notice that when Sana reduced her contact with others (perhaps in order to protect herself from the discomfort of relationships with peers who appear to have 'moved on'), she is also thwarting her future involvement in the social opportunities which might have buffered against the loneliness which she now experiences (Townsend & McWhirter, 2005). Relationships and 'group memberships' can serve as a resource, offering social capital to provide stability during times of change (Iyer et al., 2009), but can see in this example that such resources may require support and scaffolding if they are to be sustained during times of crisis.

Shifting Between Dependence and Independence

With psychosis and the changing sense of self comes a shift in the relational dynamics of many of the young people, from positions of independence to dependency, to a move towards increased independence once more:

> *Achara: Even though I moved out already, but now that I'm back at home I feel a bit more, dependent on [my mum]. … I dunno maybe it's just 'cause I'm living with my parents again so, which just feels a bit more like, I dunno, maybe it's 'cause I'm not working, maybe when I'm working it'll feel different … or maybe I should move out again, I dunno [laughs] … 'cause like, at the beginning, I did want to move out again, but these days 'cause it feels nice to help my mum, so, I don't know, but my mum, I know she wants me to live with her … it feels a bit less grown up [laughs].*

Here we can see Achara attempting to balance her own desire for independence with her desire to help her mum, and her mum's wish for Achara to remain at home, which "feels a bit less grown up". For all of the young people, re-engaging in education or employment was important, offering an avenue through which to regain their sense of autonomy outside of the family. For some of the young people, the experience of psychosis and recovery involved not only increased dependence but inter-dependence, as highlighted by Ellie:

> *I'm quite dependent on [my parents] … there's lots of dependence on them … um, but, tiny little things, I have to pick my sister up from school sometimes, so they are dependent on me in that sense 'cause they're both at work. […] I struggle to pick up my little sister sometimes … which can be quite frustrating […] for my parents, because they do depend on me, which then makes me feel under pressure, so … which is fair enough, but, but it also encourages me to actually do things.*

We can see that for Ellie, and likely many young people, there are 'pressures' involved in moving towards independence. In this example, inter-dependence is the bridge towards this; Ellie receives support from her parents, but is building up some ways in which she can reciprocate. This mutuality is 'encouraging' and Ellie frames it as beneficial for recovery. This is perhaps because it prevents the pressure from becoming too overwhelming, especially during earlier stages of recovery.

Relationship Re-appraisal and Re-evaluation

In connection with the changing sense of self, all of the young people reference a re-appraisal of their relationships with family and friends. To some extent, such re-appraisal is a common feature of the transition from adolescence into adulthood. However, for some of the young people in our study, the experience of psychosis itself had prompted a re-evaluation of the helpfulness of friendships. For example, below we can see Samuelle talking about friends, who he came to perceive as a "negative influence". He described a desire to live his life in accordance to his own values:

> *There were some friends which are too removed, obviously, umm … because […] it was a negative influence to me […] more for my […] academics and stuff… but then […] I had to umm, to, umm remove some of the friends, not remove, that's a strong word, but umm, you know, uhh, have my own path, and uhh, understanding that, you know, there are some friends that are gonna be good, and some friends that are not.*

For some, their experience of psychosis has led to an increased awareness of their mental health and wellbeing, and of those who impact upon this; Helene talks about 'cutting off' others who she feels are "triggering":

I kind of cut these people off, the ones that don't help me. ... I just, don't talk to them, really, and if there's someone who's triggering me, or something, like people from my old church, preachers and stuff, I, I have to ignore them, even though I don't want to [...] I feel like I'm being mean to them or rude to them, umm, I just need to think about my mental health [...] that was difficult because, I felt really really guilty [...] but ... I don't wanna fall in to that, back again ... it was triggering.

We can see that the re-appraisal of relationships and subsequent distancing from others who are perceived as unhelpful can be difficult, perhaps especially given that social ties and connectedness are so important for young people, and that psychosis can make relationships difficult. However, all of the young people also spoke about positive re-appraisals of relationships, as illustrated by Radhiya:

I realised [my mum] was there for me, no matter what ... before, when I was ill, I felt she was there but not all the time, but then when I went through this, it just made me realise ... [becomes tearful] ... she's there for me no matter what.

Radhiya describes in a powerful and emotive way, as did many of the young people, a new-found appreciation and gratitude for her relationship with her mum, which developed in meaning following her experience of psychosis.

The Evolution of Others' Sense-Making

Many of the young people spoke about the temporality of others' sense-making of psychosis and recovery. Some of the young people described how their families initially found the psychosis difficult to understand, and sometimes accept, with some of the young people feeling blamed by others:

Helene: When I got to hospital and the doctors explained to [my mum] that it might be, a mental health issue, think then she actually started to think, 'Okay, I need to be there for her, and, it's not her fault', basically … [she was then] more supportive, trying to calm me down, as well, and just stay strong … because she used to be angry all the time, you know, 'Stop being that way', but […] when she knew it was mental health problem, she was more patient with me as well.

We can see how Helene experienced her mum as being more supportive once her understanding of Helene's mental health difficulties developed. A similar narrative was provided by Achara, suggesting a developing appreciation of Achara's difficulties:

I feel like my mum's nicer to me [now] … [laughs] … maybe because she knows I'm going through stuff.

Such descriptions may be reflective of stigma 'processes' (Wood et al., 2015), such as moving from lack of understanding to understanding, or from judgement to non-judgement. For other young people, family were experienced as more understanding as the episode of psychosis initially unfolded, but less so currently. Sameera spoke about her earlier loss of touch with reality, and the sense that her mum equated this with an 'unaccountability':

[Mum is more strict with me now] probably because I didn't know what I was doing then, now I have no excuse.

There was a sense that some families hoped or expected that recovery would be a quicker process, or a more clearly demarcated change. For some young people, who experienced change more slowly, or less clearly, this meant that they felt that they were lagging behind the family's understanding of where they should be. Jamie experienced his family's understanding in a similar way, and spoke about how the support they give has changed over time:

I think they like ... try to give me, like ... support, from, umm ... I dunno whether to say from a distance or, like, from ... just sorta like, I dunno I think 'cause it's, they've tried and they've tried, I think they just sorta like ... you know, leaving it with me, and just, you know like ... not leaving me, not leaving me alone, to, like, let, still like, showing that they're there and stuff ... just with a text or like a call and stuff [...] 'cause they've tried and tried, racked their brains, and like ... I mean like, like, first, probably like, 9 months, like, they did understand, you know like, and they didn't push me, didn't try and motivate me to do anything ... and then like, obviously like, once I was feeling better and stuff it was just like, you know, you need to like ... only, only, only the right motivation, but, I think, just 'cause I didn't, didn't comply with it, it was just, it was causing them stress.

In Jamie's account there is a sense that his family felt increasingly desperate and perhaps exasperated in their attempts to support Jamie with his difficulties, which have developed from 'positive-' to 'negative-symptoms'. Jamie's account also highlights the temporality of others' expectations, which may increase over time and cause family 'stress' when young people are perceived as 'non-compliant' with suggestions in support of their recovery. For some young people, this resulted in an increased sense of responsibility for their own recovery:

Sana: They know they can't fix me, but they're ... trying to help me whilst I fix myself.

Re-engaging with a Reciprocal Network

Over time, the young people sought to re-engage with a reciprocal relational network, in which others are inter-connected, provide support to each other, and to which the young people wish to 'give back'. Such reciprocity may provide opportunities for 'ego-strengthening' (Huckle et al., 2021), via mechanisms of contribution and feeling valued.

Some young people utilised people in their network as a 'middle-man' between themselves and others, highlighting a web-like relational system; Jamie spoke about 'problem-solving' with his sister about how he might re-connect with his parents. Sometimes, others in the network took this role of 'middle-man' upon themselves; Ellie described how her mum spoke to one of her own friends who also has a daughter experiencing mental health problems, in order to 'set-up' a friendship between the two young people, which may be seen as mutually beneficial for Ellie's mum and Ellie.

Most of the young people spoke about the importance of reciprocity within their relationships, and a keenness to 'give back' to those who have helped and supported them through their difficult experiences. Ellie describes an emotional reciprocity and inter-dependence by which she can give back to a friend, which feels important and makes a "big difference" within her recovery, appearing to boost self-worth and sense of purpose:

> *[My friend], she's very good at sharing her problems with you but not in a way which drags you down, in a way that makes you feel like you're having an input in her life [...] like asking for your opinion on things, little things like that really help I think, they make you feel like necessary, or just like your opinion matters ... you know like, 'You can help me, it's not just like I'm gonna help you all the time' ... which, makes a big difference.*

Ellie used colour to 'group' people in her close network, using heart shapes to represent relational meaning. Some individuals included at Time 1 are not represented at Time 2 (see Fig. 9.2), whilst the relationships Ellie has with her mum and siblings appear to have developed in significance. Arrows are used to imply directionality within her relationships, inter-dependency, and reciprocity. Not only does Ellie depict her connections with others, she represents how others are connected, implying a more inter-connected and dynamic network within which Ellie is well-embedded and which has grown since Time 1.

For other young people, reciprocity was conveyed in a more transactional sense. Jamie spoke about his efforts to help others at his supported living accommodation with their endeavours to find work, and also spoke about it being important to 'exchange' effort with his family. Jamie and Ellie's descriptions of practical and emotional reciprocity, respectively, may reflect gender differences in the roles the young people are adopting,

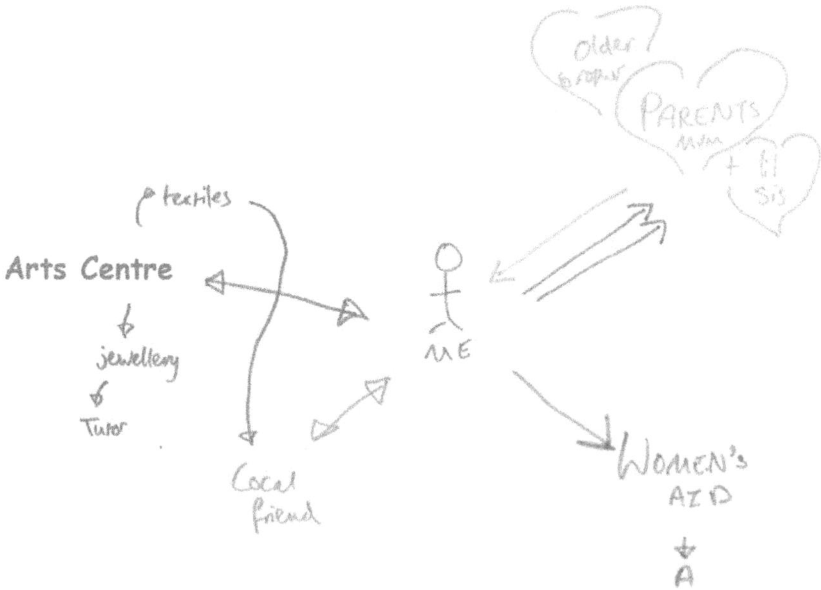

Fig. 9.2 Ellie's image at Time 2

and differing emphases placed upon 'emotional labour' and practical 'providing' within relational contexts (e.g. Kahn et al., 2011):

> *Jamie: If I get back in to the real world, and like … you know … it's like just sorta like bringing summat to the table, I don't wanna like … go there and be like a spare sheep sorta thing.*

This excerpt is one of several in which Jamie appeared regretful around not 'making an effort' with his family, as they have with him. Jamie's metaphor of himself as a "spare sheep" illuminates his view of himself as perhaps a 'spare part' or 'black sheep', which fits with his wider narrative around not contributing to the family in ways deemed acceptable by them. Jamie spoke a number of times about wishing to 'bring something to the table', which, whilst struggling to do so at the time of research, appears to represent his need to give back. We know from other research that this kind of reciprocity is highly valued by young people (e.g. see

Boden-Stuart et al., 2021) and that there are many ways in which young people can make meaningful contributions to family life during their recovery (e.g. see Allman et al., 2018). These kinds of processes may benefit from guided conversations and external support to prompt reflection and change within the family.

Reflections

The importance of positive, frequent, reciprocal connection with others during recovery from FEP is reflective of the universal human 'need to belong' (Baumeister & Leary, 1995). In these personal accounts from young people, we see a snapshot of how their relational needs and connectedness to others are experienced as dynamic. The sense of the young people's relatedness to others as evolving and transforming appears to mirror a process in relation to the young person's own sense of self. This fluctuating dynamism may be a response both to changes in life stage (Arnett, 2000) and to the puzzling changes in self-experience associated with psychosis (Humpston & Broome, 2016). It is a doubly disruptive experience for these young people.

In a sense, the most important things we might take from this, when we reflect on how best to meet the needs of young people experiencing psychosis, are firstly to be aware of how important peer relationships are for them, and secondly, to be mindful of the 'double vortex' of emerging adulthood and psychosis, which disrupts the means by which their relational needs would normally be met on two dimensions at once. In particular, we might bear in mind that, because friendships appear to be especially vulnerable to 'withering', it is important to think about how we can nurture new friendships and how we can protect and sustain existing friendships. This is a dimension of Early Intervention work which is often informal. It is under-researched as an evidence-based practiced and under-resourced as a clinical activity. It would benefit from the formal contribution of professionals in youth work and social workers.

Phenomenologically speaking, we live in worlds that we ourselves sustain. In the context of psychosis, a world which is shared with trusted others is likely to be helpful for safety and recovery. We can see, in the cases discussed here, that friendships are an important route to both reciprocity and self-reflection. These are likely to be important stepping-stones on the route to recovery for young people, and efforts to be support young people in these endeavours seem likely to be rewarded with good outcomes.

References

Allman, J., Cooke, A., Whitfield, B., & McCartney, M. (2018). "It doesn't mean I'm useless": How do young people experiencing psychosis contribute to their families and why are contributions sometimes overlooked? *Psychosis, 10*(1), 11–21. https://doi.org/10.1080/17522439.2017.1413129

Arnett, J. J. (2000). Emerging adulthood: A theory of development from the late teens through the twenties. *American Psychologist, 55*(5), 469.

Bagwell, C. L., Bender, S. E., Andreassi, C. L., Kinoshita, T. L., Montarello, S. A., & Muller, J. G. (2005). Friendship quality and perceived relationship changes predict psychosocial adjustment in early adulthood. *Journal of Social and Personal Relationships, 22*(2), 235–54.

Baugh, C., & Lucas-Motley, H. (Eds.). (2021). *Quality standards for early intervention in psychosis services.* Available at: https://www.rcpsych.ac.uk/docs/default-source/improving-care/ccqi/quality-networks/early-intervention-in-psychosis-teams-(eipn)/quality-standards-for-eip-services-2nd-edition.pdf?sfvrsn=131a6e4e_2

Baumeister, R. F., & Leary, M. R. (1995). The need to belong: Desire for interpersonal attachments as a fundamental human motivation. *Psychological Bulletin, 117*, 497-529.

Birchwood, M. (2003). Pathways to emotional dysfunction in first-episode psychosis. *The British Journal of Psychiatry: the Journal of Mental Science, 182*, 373.

Blatt, S. J., & Luyten, P. (2009). A structural–developmental psycho-dynamic approach to psychopathology: Two polarities of experience across the life span. *Development and Psychopathology, 21*, 793–814.

Boden, Z., & Eatough, V. (2014). Understanding more fully: A multimodal hermeneutic-phenomenological approach. *Qualitative Research in Psychology, 11*(2), 160–177.

Boden, Z., Larkin, M., & Iyer, M. (2018). Picturing ourselves in the world: Drawings, IPA and the Relational Mapping Interview. For a special issue on

IPA of *Qualitative Research in Psychology*. https://doi.org/10.1080/14780887.2018.1540679

Boden-Stuart, Z. V. R., Larkin, M., & Harrop, C. (2021). Young adults' dynamic relationships with their families in early psychosis: Identifying relational strengths and supporting relational agency. *Psychology and Psychotherapy: Theory, Research and Practice, 94*, 646–666. https://doi.org/10.1111/papt.12337

Cheng, F., Kirkbride, J. B., Lennox, B. R., Perez, J., Masson, K., Lawrence, K., & Jones, P. B. (2011). Administrative incidence of psychosis assessed in an early intervention service in England: First epidemiological evidence from a diverse, rural and urban setting. *Psychological Medicine, 41*, 949–958.

Cooke, A. (Ed.). (2017). *Understanding psychosis and schizophrenia*. British Psychological Society. Available at: https://www1.bps.org.uk/system/files/userfiles/Division%20of%20Clinical%20Psychology/public/CAT-1657.pdf

Crumlish, N., Whitty, P., Clarke, M., Browne, S., Kamali, M., Gervin, M., & O'Callaghan, E. (2009). Beyond the critical period: Longitudinal study of 8-year outcome in first episode non-affective psychosis. *British Journal of Psychiatry, 194*(1), 18–24.

Erikson, E. H. (Ed.). (1963). *Youth: Change and challenge*. Basic books.

Gilbert, P. (2002). Body shame: A biopsychosocial conceptualisation and overview, with treatment implications. In P. Gilbert, & J. Miles (Eds.), *Body shame: Conceptualisation, research and treatment* (pp. 3–54). London: Brunner-Routledge.

Griffiths, R., Mansell, W., Edge, D., & Tai, S. (2019). Sources of distress in first-episode psychosis: A systematic review and qualitative metasynthesis. *Qualitative Health Research, 29*(1), 107–123.

Harrop, C., & Trower, P. (2003). *Why does schizophrenia develop at late adolescence? A cognitive-developmental approach to psychosis*. Wiley.

Harrop, C., Ellett, L., Brand, R., & Lobban, F. (2014). Friends interventions in early psychosis: A narrative review and call to action. *Early Intervention in Psychiatry*. https://doi.org/10.1111/eip.12172

Huckle, C., Lemmel, F., & Johnson, S. (2021). Experiences of friendships of young people with first-episode psychosis: A qualitative study. *PLoS One, 16*(7), e0255469.

Humpston, C. S., & Broome, M. R. (2016). Perplexity. In G. Stanghellini & M. Aragona (Eds.), *An experiential approach to psychopathology*. Springer. https://doi.org/10.1007/978-3-319-29945-7_13

Iyer, A., Jetten, J., Tsivrikos, D., Postmes, T., & Haslam, S. A. (2009). The more (and more compatible) the merrier: multiple group memberships and identity compatibility as predictors of adjustment after life transitions. *British Journal of Social Psychology, 48*(4), 707–733.

Kahn, J., McGill, B., & Bianchi, S. (2011). Help to family and friends: Are there gender differences at older ages? *Journal of Marriage and the Family, 73*(1), 77–92.

Kidd, I. (2022). Loneliness and interpersonal connection. *RIP talk at UoB*. Available at: https://www.birmingham.ac.uk/news/2022/cal-ptr-loneliness-and-mental-health

Kirova, A., & Emme, M. (2006). Using photography as a means of phenomenological seeing: "Doing phenomenology" with immigrant children. *Indo-Pacific Journal of Phenomenology, 6*(sup1), 1–12.

Leamy, M., Bird, V., Le Boutillier, C., Williams, J., & Slade, M. (2011). Conceptual framework for personal recovery in mental health: Systematic review and narrative synthesis. *The British Journal of Psychiatry, 199*(6), 445–452.

Levula, A., Wilson, A., & Harré, M. (2016). The association between social network factors and mental health at different life stages. *Quality of Life Research, 25*(7), 1725–1733.

Lim, M. H., & Gleeson, J. F. (2014). Social connectedness across the psychosis spectrum: Current issues and future directions for interventions in loneliness. *Frontiers in Psychiatry, 5*, 154.

Linszen, D., & Birchwood, M. (2000). The early phase of psychosis and schizophrenia: A critical period for patients, families and the profession. In M. Birchwood, D. Fowler, & C. Jackson (Eds.), *Early intervention in psychosis: A guide to concepts, evidence and interventions* (pp. 261–277). Wiley.

Macdonald, E. M., Hayes, R. L., & Baglioni A, J. (2000). The quantity and quality of the social networks of young people with early psychosis compared with closely matched controls. *Schizophrenia Research, 46*, 25–30.

Mann, F., Bone, J. K., Lloyd-Evans, B., Frerichs, J., Pinfold, V., Ma, R., Wang, J., & Johnson, S. (2017). A life less lonely: The state of the art in interventions to reduce loneliness in people with mental health problems. *Social Psychiatry and Psychiatric Epidemiology, 52*(6), 627–638.

Matthews, T., Danese, A., Caspi, A., Fisher, H. L., Goldman-Mellor, S., Kepa, A., et al. (2018). Lonely young adults in modern Britain: Findings from an epidemiological cohort study. *Psychological Medicine*, 1–10.

McNamara, N., Coyne, I., Ford, T., Paul, M., Singh, S., & McNicholas, F. (2017). Exploring social identity change during mental healthcare transition. *European Journal of Social Psychology, 47*, 889–903.

Moretti, M. M., & Peled, M. (2004). Adolescent-parent attachment: Bonds that support healthy development. *Pediatrics & Child Health, 9*(8), 551–555.

Motta, V. N., & Larkin, M. (2022). Absence of other and disruption of self: An interpretative phenomenological analysis of the meaning of loneliness in the context of life in a religious community. *Phenomenology and the Cognitive Sciences, 22*, 55. https://doi.org/10.1007/s11097-022-09832-8

NICE. (2014). *Psychosis and schizophrenia in adults: Prevention and management.* Retrieved from https://www.nice.org.uk/guidance/cg178?unlid=906847162201611420233l

NHS Choices. (2019, December 10). *Psychosis.* Available at: http://www.nhs.uk/conditions/Psychosis/Pages/Introduction.aspx. Retrieved 2 Feb 2022.

Schön, U. K., Denhov, A., & Topor, A. (2009). Social relationships as a decisive factor in recovering from severe mental illness. *The International Journal of Social Psychiatry, 55*(4), 336–347.

Smith, J. A., Flowers, P., & Larkin, M. (2012). *Interpretative phenomenological analysis: Theory, method and research.* SAGE.

Tew, J., Ramon, S., Slade, M., Bird, V., Melton, J., & Le Boutillier, C. (2012). Social factors and recovery from mental health difficulties: A review of the evidence. *British Journal of Social Work, 42*, 443–460. https://doi.org/10.1093/bjsw/bcr076

Thornicroft, G., Rose, D., & Kassam, A. (2007). Discrimination in health care against people with mental illness. *International Review of Psychiatry, 19*, 113–122.

Townsend, K. C., & McWhirter, B. T. (2005). Connectedness: A review of the literature with implications for counseling, assessment, and research. *Journal of Counseling & Development, 83*(2), 191–201.

Van Harmelen, A. L., Kievit, R. A., Ioannidis, K., Neufeld, S., Jones, P. B., Bullmore, E., Dolan, R., The NSPN Consortium., Fonagy, F., & Goodyer, I. (2017). Adolescent friendships predict later resilient functioning across psychosocial domains in a healthy community cohort. *Psychological medicine, 47*(13), 2312–2322.

Windell, D., & Norman, R. M. (2012). A qualitative analysis of influences on recovery following a first episode of psychosis. *International Journal of Social Psychiatry, 59*(5), 493–500.

Wood, L., Burke, E., Byrne, R., Pyle, M., Chapman, N., & Morrison, A. (2015). Stigma in psychosis: A thematic synthesis of current qualitative evidence. *Psychosis, 7*(2), 152–165.

Woodman, E., & McArthur, M. (2017). Young people's experiences of family connectedness: Supporting social work practice with families and young people. *The British Journal of Social Work, 48*, 693.

10

Hunger Trauma, Relational Care and Emergency Food Support

Carl Walker, Orly Klein, Hilary Schan, Brian Devlin, Mary Wise, and Dani Plowman

Hunger, Suffering and Care Ethics

If we understand wellbeing as a state of affairs that involves a transaction between individuals and supportive relationships and environments (Stokols, 2003), then the nature of care ethics and practices becomes relevant. We understand wellbeing and distress to be relational, social and economically and politically mediated. It is useful here to draw upon an empirical ethics of care (Pols, 2015) that allows for an analysis of plural and conflicting notions of 'good care', rather than to constitute normative 'good practice' in care. Certain spaces, relations, institutions and

C. Walker (✉) • O. Klein
University of Brighton, Brighton, UK
e-mail: c.j.walker@brighton.ac.uk

H. Schan • B. Devlin • M. Wise
Worthing Food Foundation, Worthing, UK

D. Plowman
West Sussex County Council, Chichester, UK

Z. Boden-Stuart, M. Larkin (eds.), *Relationships and Mental Health*,
https://doi.org/10.1007/978-3-031-50047-3_10

circumstances enable equivocal care practices to emerge. Pols' empirical ethics of care makes it possible to analyse the different and sometimes conflicting notions of what is good care. Within care, practices and relations foreground some elements of care and marginalise others.

In the context of food insecurity, research suggests that different experiences of care and support shape people's experiences not only of care encounters but also of themselves and who they are. When people come to a foodbank they enter the unknown and open themselves up to forms of scrutiny from others that they may never have experienced before (Crooks & Evans, 2007). This can induce anxiety and uncertainty as well as real, grounded concerns over whether revealing their lack of food will have implications for their ability to look after their dependents. Much of the previous research into food insecurity has outlined the psychological consequences of hunger in terms of individualised common mental health terms, such as depression, anxiety and suicidal ideation. We believe, however, that to understand the psychosocial experience of food insecurity in such terms risks undermining the wider structural antecedents of the distress of hunger and risks misrepresenting a very distinct experience of trauma. The research makes clear that 'hunger trauma' leads to very specific feelings of emotional distress, shame and guilt while also affecting people's sense of identity and status. Framing the distress associated with hunger through the lens of 'trauma' resonates with the 'Power Threat Meaning Framework' (Johnstone et al., 2018) which draws on a trauma-informed approach. Where distress is shaped by specific sets of economic, social and political arrangements often beyond the proximal experiences of those who are living through hunger.

In the UK, the welfare state is shrinking and the cost of living is increasing. The Environment, Food and Rural Affairs Committee suggested that nearly 6 million adults and 1.7 million children were struggling to get enough food between September 2020 and February 2021. This accords to 11.5% of the UK population. For some, receiving any kind of charitable support, but especially food support, reinforces the social and moral authority of the caregiver over the care receiver (Parsell & Clarke, 2020). There is inbuilt humiliation and power imbalance involved in charity use. The increasing number of faith-based providers as social service providers may also have specific impacts on how people experience food support encounters. The shame of charity adds a layer to the shame of those failing to experience economic success and is a reason that charity has been described as an act of virtue *and* oppression (Parsell & Clarke, 2020).

This chapter focuses on the experiences of using emergency food support organisations and the forms of psychosocial trauma endured by many forced into food support. We explore food support organisations as sites of relational care that foreground the notion of charitable support as an act of both virtue *and* oppression.

The Research

Participants from foodbanks across the Adur and Worthing Food Network were invited to take part in in-depth interviews for this research. Eighteen people, all of whom regularly used emergency food support, took part from four different foodbanks. Of the participants, 3 were male and 15 were female. All participants were over 18. Interviews explored experiences of accessing and attaining emergency food support and the way that hunger and the use of emergency food support impacted physical and mental wellbeing. Data was analysed using thematic analysis, a flexible analytic method (Braun & Clarke, 2008) that allows researchers to identify, analyse and report patterns within qualitative data. Ethics approval was given by the University of Brighton College Research Ethics Committee and all names are pseudonyms.

Findings

What is clear from the data collected through these interviews is that the psychosocial experience of using emergency food support is complex and multifaceted. The psychological consequences of hunger are often understood through mental health terms such as depression, anxiety and suicidal ideation as well as experiences with a social element, such as shame and humiliation. We believe that this way of framing food insecurity compartmentalises and risks artificially reducing a traumatic experience which is also intrinsically political, economic, discursive, relational and embodied. Moreover, if we are to understand the most effective ways to help people needing food support, it may be useful to discuss the complexity of hunger trauma as a distinct and complex set of experiences.

The embodied experience of hunger in individuals and families defies a simple psychological reading of 'mental health', instead revealing a cycle of trauma that is as much social and economic as it is psychological. Being forced to access food support manifests a set of experiences that are to some extent distinct in nature from other experiences of trauma.

Here we present five themes drawn from our study, and then discuss these through a relational lens, in order to consider what a more caring approach to food support might look like.

The Unavoidable Desperation of Hidden Hunger

In a theme reflected in *all* of the interviews, participants spoke of turning to food support in desperation, as they found themselves with no other options. For example, Erin described a set of circumstances including illness, changes in job status, the failure of the furlough scheme and a social security net that didn't cover her costs. This meant that her family required access to the foodbank. Paula described a similar convergence of circumstances beyond her control:

> *It was being a single parent, it was erm … being made redundant, then erm … just, yeah, just being on the breadline, getting no maintenance from ex-partners, that sort of thing. Everything that's attached to single motherhood, really. It was all when I had my third baby.* (Paula)

It was notable that these circumstances did not arise from the participants' poor judgement but from life events outside of their control, and their effects were disproportionately experienced by, and managed by, women.

The Constant Crisis

One of the key features that moves people from food insecurity to food support is the relentless grinding nature of living in constant crisis. For some, it means not sleeping. It means regularly breaking down in tears and for some, below, much worse. But the key element that people highlighted was the constant and enduring nature of feeling like your life is in crisis and you've lost control.

This sense of desperation and worry, and the cumulative impact of these financial stressors, can have different impacts on people in hunger. A key element shared by all was the constant, grinding nature of living in hunger and the inability to find relief or to escape:

> *It feels like the sky falling down on top of you when you realise that I can't, I'm in Council Tax arrears, I'm in arrears with my with my gas and my electricity, you know, when you can't buy your kids school shoes, you can't buy them, you know, new school clothes, you can't buy them, you know, and everything has gone. And, you know, you just think, oh, God, you know, what do I do?* (Sue)

The Shame of Hunger

In *The Politics of Trauma*, Haines (2019) notes that there is a social and economic distribution of dignity, safety and belonging. Those on lower incomes and living in food poverty find themselves subject to a range of stigmatising representations of their lives. Poverty is often dismissed as self-inflicted, and the shame of poverty happens when we feel a failure or lack in the eyes of others. People living in poverty are tortured by the fear of shame and not meeting others' expectations. The accompanying real and imagined social rejection can feed onto the trauma of hunger (Hudson, 2015).

Food insecurity has many public markers that can be identified by family and friends. Hunger is a trauma that can shatter people's sense of wellbeing and can feel like a loss of security, sense of order and can result in social rejection (Hudson, 2015). Some can be prepared to go to the most extreme lengths to evade the shame and stigma of hunger. Here,

Helen's daughter is prepared to go hungry rather than expose herself as needing free school meals, let alone food support:

> You know, she literally went all day without any food, didn't tell me, and it's only the fact I got an email saying, 'your daughter did not come and collect her lunch', because she's embarrassed by it you know, the thought of having to go to a foodbank is even worse. She said you know, "I'm glad mummy, that they come here", she said, "because people probably think we're just getting shopping delivered", because she is so embarrassed by it. I mean I haven't admitted it to a lot of people, I've told my vicar but that is about it because I'm embarrassed you know, I don't want to be in this situation.

Food and the social practices around food are fundamental components of our identity, the way we see ourselves and the ways in which others see us. Social identity is the way that we orientate ourselves to the social world. Many of us have different identities depending on which areas of our lives we are orienting to and which people we are interacting with. Having the choice to express yourself through a particular identity allows us to navigate often very different social settings and social pressures. In this context identity choice is an important part of wellbeing. Experiences like those above where people are forced through destitution to expose their hunger markers publicly minimise their ability to present themselves in public in favourable ways. These markers have relational consequences. For example, Sally notes the challenges of being a visible user of a foodbank and describes the challenge of hiding the shame of foodbank reliance on children:

> Yeah, so my youngest is 6 and I've got a 12-year-old daughter, nearly 13, and I've got a 14-year-old son. And the oldest two, they're like, you know, they don't, they don't want to be having foodbanks. They erm …, you know, they don't want that, because they're aware of it. So everything's, everything's highly visible and when you're trying to hide things and crack through it, it's a, you feel a bit too visible.

In this scenario, where identity is fixed and enforced, people will make often extreme choices not to expose this identity. Not least because identity loss or enforced identities can be experienced as catastrophic (Haslam et al., 2012). Being excluded from acceptable cultural food practices means being unable to meet social expectations and these social aspects of food are recognised as important, not least because food provides a sense of normality and routine for people (O'Connell & Brannen, 2021). When these routines become shameful, it can have long-term impacts on identity.

Food as a Relational Commitment

For our participants, the choosing, providing, preparing and sharing of food all had important personal and relational functions which were lost when poverty left them hungry. Derek outlines the impact of not being able to provide for his partner, something that had been central to his identity through his life and left him with a feeling of deep inadequacy:

> *I felt like I was inadequate, I suppose, is the word, I couldn't provide for my partner and myself, I've worked all my life from, since leaving school I've been working.* (Derek)

Part of the social element of food is about being able to engage in important cultural food rituals. Being able to rehearse these rituals during a period of sustained loss of status can be profoundly supportive and enabling, as Pippa illustrates here:

> *Yeah, it was a real, yeah, it just really, really helped. It came to the point, I think, that it was normal again, you know, because instead of having tinned veg or frozen veg, we were all prepping it together, which we always do at Christmas, you know, so it was nice.* (Pippa)

One of the difficult elements of food support is the dehumanising aspect of losing control of what you chose to eat. Below, Pat notes the impact of others controlling what you eat:

I mean I do try to make things like from scratch using these tinned tomatoes so yeah, I suppose it does. I mean the tins of soup we're not really big soup eaters apart from tomato soup. So, I think if you just rely on it it's, you know, it does kind of control what you eat. (Pat)

Reneging on a perceived relational commitment can have consequences for the self. In the context of these relational aspects of hunger, it was notable that one way in which food support impacts upon identity is through pervasive experiences of guilt. Participants spoke of experiencing multiple forms of concurrent guilt with regards to people they felt they were letting down. Experiences of guilt and humiliation took on a particular shape in the context of parenting, where parents had internalised the experience of poverty and reported feeling that they had failed as a parent since they were unable to access one of the central hallmarks of being able to understand themselves as a 'good parent'—that of being able to provide for their children. For example:

I felt very anxious, and I really felt like I'd failed as a parent, to provide for my son, to have to look for external support, it really did feel like I was a total let-down as a mother. (Louise)

I mean, everything is so expensive, you know, and for me it's constant guilt with my children, you know, not giving them that lifestyle that they deserve. (Sally)

Some spoke of the pervasive feeling of guilt being a constant presence in their lives. Each new financial challenge evoked a further iteration of shame and guilt.

The Indignity of Food Support

Participants described various ways in which the relational structures and interactions involved in seeking food support threatened their identities and dignity. Research suggests that different experiences of care and support shape people's experiences not only of care encounters but also of themselves and who they are (Pols, 2015). When people come to a foodbank they enter the unknown and open themselves up to forms of scrutiny that they may never have experienced before (Crooks & Evans, 2007). This can induce anxiety and uncertainty as well as grounded concerns over whether revealing their lack of food will have implications for their ability to look after their dependents. Liminal spaces in society are spaces where people transition from one way of understanding themselves to another, and foodbanks can act as a liminal space where people transition from independent, autonomous self-supporting individuals to 'clients' or, worse, 'scroungers' depending on the messages received during these food support encounters. For some, receiving any kind of charitable support, but especially food support, reinforces the social and moral authority of the caregiver over the care receiver (Parsell & Clarke, 2020).

Reciprocation is important. Accepting a gift, without reciprocating, is to show subordination (Parsell & Clarke, 2020). In order to stop denying a person the status of 'full partner' in a social interaction, providing opportunities to give is crucially important when people are forced into circumstances where they feel they need to 'take'. Foodbanks are spaces that can be shaped, controlled and moulded so that experiences of humiliation are minimised and experiences of dignified autonomy are amplified. Every gesture and conversation between those providing and those seeking support can be crucial. But a key element is also the nuts and bolts of practices around food choice, reciprocity, food delivery and whether or not a service has a referral process.

The foodbank sector is largely unregulated and this can contribute to a deeply problematic overlap between supporting those in need and the desire to indulge in religious evangelism. For example, Helen here outlines the challenges of religious moralising and judgement in a foodbank that was run by a religious institution:

> *It's the stigma and it's the where do you get the voucher from and then it's, there's a certain element to them of trying to convert you and pull you into their way of thinking and praying and I bloody pray and it's none of your business. You know, I'm not here to pray, I'm, you know, I'm here to get the basic of basic food so I stopped going.* (Helen)

Another issue, illustrated by Sam, is the issue of a foodbank infrastructure that facilitates public judgement of others. Some foodbanks use a queuing system which feels exposing, anxiety-provoking and shaming for those who need emergency support. This infrastructure can also be enacted via relational interactions with food providers, as Sam demonstrates:

> *I think the whole idea that you have to queue up to get something so personal to you [...] Is somebody going to phone my daughter and say, I've seen your mum at the foodbank queue? [...] And I don't know if it's just me, it might be just me, but I just wasn't comfortable with the whole experience at all and I would avoid it. Sam.*
>
> *They had it all out on the table and she said, 'Pick what you want.' So, I went to pick up a pack of four burgers or something like that and she said, oh no, that's for families and took it back off my hand. Well, I nearly bloody died, I was mortified, and she literally snapped it out of my hand. And I remember okay, I'm never doing this again and I cried all the way home from Victoria Road to here.* (Sam)

In both of these examples, Sam describes choosing hunger over shame ('I'm never doing this again', 'I would avoid it'). People can be dehumanised by systems and structures of food support (Chase & Walker, 2012) and often attempt to avoid shame by withdrawing from social interactions. This can lead to a sense of powerlessness and an attendant physical and psychological deterioration.

Relational Opportunities for Dignity

A key element in dignified food support is to have a clear focus on protecting every encounter and creating a culture of care that foregrounds dignity and humanising practices. Research suggests that eating is an intensely personal act because what we eat communicates to others our beliefs, cultural and social backgrounds and experiences (Culture Decanted, 2014). The social aspects of food are recognised as important and food engenders a sense of normality for people (O'Connell &

Brannen, 2021). Where one gets food has important social, psychological, economic and political contexts (Vissing & Gu, 2017).

Obtaining food from a farmer's market, restaurant, neighbourhood corner shop, grocers, petrol station convenience shop or grandma's house, all have different economic, psychological and social dimensions for the person giving, and receiving, the food. People acquire an identity not just from what they eat, but from where and how they get the food. When people do not have enough to eat through customary avenues, they may seek assistance from emergency food support organisations and this involves a public acknowledgement of one's impoverished or marginalised status (Vissing & Gu, 2017). People may use a variety of strategies to mask the fact that they can't afford food; saving face disguises the embarrassment of admitting that one is hungry.

People have many different pathways into hunger trauma and the complexity of these pathways resists a top-down, bureaucratic approach to emergency food provision. There are complex social dynamics that play out in any food acquisition system, raising a range of important considerations for physical wellbeing and also mental health (Cannuscio et al., 2010). The emotions people feel when going to ask for food include anger, frustration, shame and resentment (Vissing, 1996). Their embarrassment, frustration and confusion about how to self-advocate while feeling vulnerable is an interaction problem for both them and those who are in the position of providing them food. Those seeking food support frequently experience profound anxiety and desperation that leaves them unable to focus on a range of goals due to the immediate need to organise food for themselves and/or their family. The move to reach out for food support can feel intensely shameful and undignified. This desperation, together with a mistrust of what other people and organisations will make of the need for food support, means that food support encounters must be nuanced and carefully protected.

However, class-based differences often exist in emergency food support organisations between those who volunteer and run emergency food support and those who use the services. Indeed, many who run emergency food support organisations are well-meaning, middle-class providers and may have a different understanding of the health, emotional and social needs of service users (Vissing & Gu, 2017). One reason hypothesised for potential staff insensitivity reflected social class bias; the majority of patrons at the food support are visibly poor and/or homeless, while those serving them tended to be middle class. Being unaware of the user's lived experiences is not uncommon for support organisations to intentionally or inadvertently engage in interactions that do not dignify those who are asking for help (Vissing & Gu, 2017).

Good intentions do not necessarily result in good communications. How food support users feel treated influences their self-esteem and their desire to return or use future services. When people visit food pantries, often they seek both food and solace, but Vissing and Gu (2017) suggest that, too often, they receive too little of both. If nuanced and carefully protected, food support can provide a level of stability, a sense of mattering and a humanising impulse that alleviates some of the trauma, builds trust and can provide the basis for relationships, further possibilities, support and signposting. Practices that allow food support users to retain control and status, such as giving back and donating food to the foodbank, or allowing parents to be the parent who brings happiness again, can have such a profound effect on the status and identity of the food support user:

> *It's obviously freed me up some finances which I would had to have spent on especially on the toiletries and her Tampax and things like that, and it's freed up things so obviously she needs things for school and that so it gives me that, just gives me that little extra not, without having to worry about things, you know, her things, so she needs to go out with her friends at the weekend. Rather than me saying oh, I haven't got the money, you know, I've got that odd few quid now where I can give her a couple of quid so she can get herself some lunch if she's out with her chums and that on a Saturday or something, you know, don't have to be embarrassing opening up a sandwich in a bag or something, you know, things like that. So it is, the impact's all positive and when it does come she loves having a look to see what we've got as well. It's almost like, you know, not knowing what you're going to get is almost as exciting as getting it, if you know what I mean, you just don't, you know.* (Dani)

Charities, where possible, need to enable reciprocity so people are seen beyond their vulnerabilities and misrecognised position to foster opportunities for reciprocal care that fosters social solidarity. Opportunities for reciprocity should be embraced by food support organisations putting dignity at the heart of their encounters.

> *So I donated all my kids' clothes to other people who are struggling, I found out who's really struggling, and I said, "Would you like a bag of girls' clothes", because I've had to ask. Sorry, you can't ask for something if you can't give something back, if you know what I mean, and that's what I try and do. I try to help somebody else, then I feel, I don't feel bad when I've had to ask.* (Tara)

> *No, well often I give him a big bag back and say, "Can you just say I'm very grateful but I don't want them to waste", so like before I knew it I had like 40 tins of soup, you know, which I make my own soup and we all have it with some crunchy bread or something, so I said, "Can I send this and give it to somebody else?" so yeah, that's what I've done, I've just given it back rather than waste it, but then it kind of looks like you're going, oh you know, I don't want that [laughs].* (Don)

Subtle practices oriented around protecting dignity can make a difference to those experiencing food support. In this quote Paula foregrounds the importance of encounters that feel relaxed, informal and non-judgemental:

> *I think they're quite erm … I think they know that it's a little bit erm …, I don't know if stigma's the right word, but they know, they don't advertise it, you know. They just, you know, say who's there and they say it's the community hub. And then when I get down, they're already halfway to the car and just giving you a wave, you know, that kind of thing. They don't make a big fuss about it, like, which is really, I don't think I'd mind, you know. I'm a bit thick skinned, anyway, when it comes to some things, so I don't think I'd mind if they stayed and had a chat, you know.* (Paula)

The section above shows just how important the human encounters in foodbanks can be in structuring not only whether people feel enabled to reach out for support but in terms of how they come to understand themselves and the trauma of living lives marred by persistent hunger.

Gendered Hunger

It should be noted that the majority of respondents who took part in this research were women. This should not come as any surprise, as research consistently shows that women are at particular risk of food insecurity and that households with children headed by single women are more likely to be food insecure (Alaimo et al., 1998). Moreover, research suggests that women are likely to make choices in regard to their own food consumption that disproportionately adversely affect them, as they seek to protect children and privilege men in the household (Power et al., 2018).

We saw in our own research references to 'guilt', not being able to provide as a mother 'what they deserve', as well as the transition into single parenthood being the catalyst for also transitioning into food insecurity. To juggle often multiple caring responsibilities, many women will work in non-standard employment, particularly low-income, part-time work (Aassve et al., 2006). Structural adjustments in the labour market and in particular the growth of the 'gig economy' have meant that much of this work has become less secure, non-standard and difficult to improve on (Rubery & Raffertey, 2013). In addition, much of women's contribution to society goes socially unrecognised, since it is unpaid. The gender-based division of labour between unpaid and paid labour renders women economically and socially more insecure and vulnerable not only to chronic poverty but also to transient poverty that can result from familial, personal or social and economic crises. These are likely drivers of the number of women using food support locally and hence experiencing disproportionate hunger trauma.

It is important to note that the use of foodbanks by women extends beyond their need to provide food for themselves or their children. Foodbanks are also important sources of other items such as nappies and menstrual products. Research suggests that it is not as widely known that foodbanks provide these items (Boyers et al., 2022) and therefore more specific outreach to women experiencing period poverty, as well as hunger, may be necessary on the part of food organisations.

Concluding Thoughts

Hunger trauma is complex and multifaceted. Those seeking food support frequently experience profound anxiety and desperation that leaves them unable to focus on a range of goals due to the immediate need to organise food for themselves and/or their family. The move to reach out for food support can feel intensely shameful and undignified. The realisation that you are struggling to feed yourself and/or family is profoundly debilitating, as is relinquishing control of your food supply to an external agency. This desperation, together with a mistrust of what other people and organisations will make of the need for food support, means that food support encounters must be nuanced and carefully protected.

Identity and status challenges are a central component of the shame, indignity and suffering associated with hunger trauma and are central to the wellbeing of foodbank users. How people are related to during these challenging encounters are profoundly important in relation to their own sense of self and status, and building new social identities can be central to recovery from trauma (Haslam et al., 2012).

The relational care that people feel when interacting with emergency food support influences their self-esteem and their desire to return or use future services. Developing interaction strategies that preserve dignity and empower individuals is part of creating humanity in society. If nuanced and carefully protected, food support can provide a level of stability, a sense of mattering and a humanising impulse that alleviates some of the trauma, builds trust and can provide the basis for relationships, further possibilities, support and signposting.

This chapter suggests that we need to note the way that support is administered and organised, to promote opportunities for reciprocity and dignity and to remove dehumanising referral processes and barriers, in order to avoid compounding, exacerbating or activating hunger trauma and to support people effectively. We recommend that food partnerships and networks not only focus on food supply but also recognise the scale and nature of hunger trauma and how it impacts their practices to minimise stigma and amplify dignified encounters. It is crucial that we recognise the identity aspirations of those who are distressed and traumatised.

While this work is focused on emergency food organisations, providers, food networks and commissioners, it would be remiss not to recognise the broad economic drivers of hunger trauma. Emergency food support and the distress inherent to those who need that support are driven by specific economic choices that maintain wealth inequalities while failing to equip a growing number of people with wages and benefits that match living costs. In these circumstances, the complex psychosocial distress around hunger trauma, and the relational care challenges that it presents, will continue to proliferate.

References

Aassve, A., Burgess, S., Propper, C., & Dickson, M. (2006). Employment, family union and childbearing decisions in Great Britain. *Journal of the Royal Statistical Society, Series A: Statistics in Society, 169*, 781–804.

Alaimo, K., Briefel, R. R., Frongillo, E. A., & Olson, C. M. (1998). Food insufficiency exists in the United States: Results from the third national health and nutrition examination survey (NHANES III). *American Journal of Public Health, 88*(3), 419–426.

Boyers, M., Garikipati, S., Biggane, A., Douglas, E., Hawkes, N., et al. (2022). Period poverty: The perceptions and experiences of impoverished women living in an inner-city area of Northwest England. *PLOS ONE, 17*(7), e0269341. https://doi.org/10.1371/journal.pone.0269341

Braun, V., & Clarke, V. (2008). Using thematic analysis in psychology. *Qualitative Research in Psychology, 3*(2), 77–101.

Cannuscio, C. C., Weiss, E. E. & Asch, D. A. (2010). The Contribution of Urban Foodways to Health Disparities. *Journal of urban health, 87*(3), 381–393.

Chase, E., & Walker, R. (2012). The co-construction of shame in the context of poverty: Beyond a threat to the social bond. *Sociology, 47*(4), 739–754.

Crooks, V. A., & Evans, J. (2007). The writings on the wall: Decoding the interior space of the hospital waiting room. In A. Williams (Ed.), *Therapeutic landscapes*. Ashgate.

Culture Decanted. (2014). *Eating yourself: We consume identity through food.* Retrieved July 16, 2022, https://culturedecanted.com/2014/10/19/eating-yourself-we-consume-identity-through-food/

Haines, S. (2019). *The politics of trauma*. North Atlantic Books.
Haslam, C., Jetten, J., & Haslam, S. A. (2012). Advancing the social cure. In *The social cure*.
Hudson, N. (2015). The trauma of poverty as social identity. *International Perspectives on Stress & Coping, 21*(2), 111–123.
Johnstone, L. & Boyle, M. with Cromby, J., Dillon, J., Harper, D., Kinderman, P., Longden, E., Pilgrim, D. & Read, J. (2018). *The Power Threat Meaning Framework: Towards the identification of patterns in emotional distress, unusual experiences and troubled or troubling behaviour, as an alternative to functional psychiatric diagnosis*. British Psychological Society. https://www1.bps.org.uk/system/files/user-files/Division%20of%20Clinical%20Psychology/public/INF299%20PTM%20Main%20web.pdf
O'Connell, R., & Brannen, J. (2021). *Families and food in hard times*. UCL Press.
Parsell, C., & Clarke, A. (2020). Charity and shame: Towards reciprocity. *Social Problems*, 1017.
Pols, J. (2015). Towards an empirical ethics in care: Relations with technologies in Health care. *Medical Health Care and Philosophy, 18*, 81–90.
Power, M., Small, N., Doherty, B., & Pickett, K. E. (2018). Hidden hunger? Experiences of food insecurity amongst Pakistani and White British women. *British Food Journal, 120*(11), 2716–2732. https://doi.org/10.1108/BFJ-06-2018-0342
Rubery, G., & Raffertey, A. (2013). Women and recession revisited. *Work, Employment and Society, 27*, 414–432.
Stokols, D., Grzywacz, J. G., McMahan, S., & Phillips, K. (2003, Sep-Oct). Increasing the health promotive capacity of human environments. *Am J Health Promot, 18*(1), 4–13. https://doi.org/10.4278/0890-1171-18.1.4. PMID: 13677958.
Vissing, Y. M. (1996). *Out of Sight, Out of Mind: Homeless Children in Small Town America*. University of Kentucky Press. Lexington, KY.
Vissing, Y., & Gu, A. J. (2017). Preserving dignity in the face of hunger: A study of food pantry utilization. *Humanity and Society, 41*(4), 461. https://doi.org/10.1177/0160597617733623

Part IV

Love and Sex: Negotiating Intimacies in Mental Health Settings

11

Implicating the Institution: Who Is Responsible for Sexuality-Related Silence in Mental Health Settings?

Kristi Urry

There is a well-established and ongoing need to improve the way that sexuality, sexual expression, and relationships are addressed in mental health settings. Existing research has tended to focus on mental health clinicians' knowledge, comfort, and competence in relation to sexuality. This approach positions the problem as a deficit in clinicians themselves, requiring interventions that act directly on that deficit. Yet, despite development of such interventions, clinicians continue to be embarrassed, avoidant, and inadequately educated in relation to sexuality (Berger-Meron et al., 2021; Higgins et al., 2008; Quinn et al., 2018; Zatloff et al., 2020); and individuals' sexuality-related needs continue to be inadequately addressed in mental health settings globally (e.g., McCann et al., 2019). In this chapter, I implicate the wider institution(s) of medicine, psychiatry, and psychology in (what I call) sexuality-related silence within mental health care and settings. I draw on my own work and a small body of existing literature to argue that effective and sustained change in

K. Urry (✉)
University of Adelaide, Adelaide, Australia
e-mail: kristi.urry@adelaide.edu.au

Z. Boden-Stuart, M. Larkin (eds.), *Relationships and Mental Health*,
https://doi.org/10.1007/978-3-031-50047-3_11

sexuality-related practice within mental health settings will not be achieved if the institutional context of clinical practice continues to be discounted. Specifically, I demonstrate the utility of shifting the locus of responsibility for sexuality-related silence from clinicians themselves to the broader institutions in which clinicians learn and work. This shift generates a range of possibilities and opportunities for understanding and addressing sexuality-related silence in mental healthcare, and I outline three broad areas for further critical examination to this end.

The arguments presented in this chapter are grounded primarily in a critical (health) psychological framework and social constructionist approach. From this perspective, health and illness are complex social phenomena that are embedded in a broader social, cultural, political, and historical context (Murray, 2015). This means that the way that we respond to health and illness—at the levels of experience, social interaction, and organised social structures including professional healthcare systems—is similarly shaped by and reflective of social processes that are specific to the sociocultural and historical context where they are unfolding. Aligned with this, I orient to the central role of language in building and making sense of our world, including health, illness, and healthcare (Burr, 2015). Drawing on these frameworks and poststructural understandings, institutions (i.e., of medicine, psychiatry, and psychology) can be usefully conceptualised as systems of knowledge that (re)produce and reinforce shared systems of meaning—or discourses—that structure our society and everyday lives (Lupton, 2012; McFarland, 2015; Weedon, 1997). Institutions also shape the way that healthcare providers navigate and respond to phenomena in their everyday practice. I draw on a theory of professional socialisation to articulate this process as it is relevant to sexuality-related care in mental health settings.

These theoretical and methodological frameworks also underpin my doctoral work, which I draw on throughout this chapter (Urry et al., 2019, 2022). In this research, I used an exploratory qualitative design to examine Australian mental health clinicians' perceptions of sexuality and sexual health. Twenty-two mental health clinicians volunteered to participate in in-depth interviews. Participants belonged to one of three disciplines (psychology, psychiatry, and mental health nursing) and were working in four Australian cities across a range of settings including inpatient, outpatient, and private. I generated several reflexive thematic analyses using this dataset (see Urry, 2020), including the two analyses discussed in this chapter.

Sexuality in Mental Healthcare: What and Why?

Sexuality (and sexual health) is a complex concept with shifting meanings depending on when, where, and why it is being discussed and by who (Burr, 2015; Epstein & Mamo, 2017; Weeks, 2010). In the context of mental distress and professional mental healthcare, a useful way to approach sexuality and sexual health is through an affirmative, holistic, and rights-based lens such as the one put forward by the World Health Organization (WHO). The WHO (2006) defines sexual health as

> a state of physical, emotional, mental and social well-being in relation to sexuality; it is not merely the absence of disease, dysfunction or infirmity. Sexual health requires a positive and respectful approach to sexuality and sexual relationships, as well as the possibility of having pleasurable and safe sexual experiences, free of coercion, discrimination and violence. For sexual health to be attained and maintained, the sexual rights of all persons must be respected, protected and fulfilled.

Importantly, this definition of sexual health is dependent on "a broad consideration of sexuality", defined as "a central aspect of being human throughout life encompasses sex, gender identities and roles, sexual orientation, eroticism, pleasure, intimacy and reproduction" (WHO, 2006). Sexuality is therefore not separable from, and even encompasses, sexual health (also see Epstein & Mamo, 2017); it is for this reason that I refer primarily to *sexuality* throughout this chapter.

Taking up this broad conceptual lens, sexuality is relevant and important in the context of professional mental healthcare for several interconnected reasons. The first and most important reason is because people who experience mental distress and access mental health services (henceforth, consumers[1]) *tell us* that sexuality, intimacy, and sexual expression are important to them (e.g., Deegan, 1999; McCann et al., 2019; White et al., 2021). Consumers' reported sexuality-related experiences and needs are wide ranging, including—but always expanding beyond—dimensions related to biological risk and safety (McCann et al., 2019). This reinforces the relevance of a holistic and affirmative approach to sexuality in the context of mental health settings and research, rather than a risk-oriented approach that prioritises biological dimensions of sexual health such as (risk of) sexually transmitted infections and blood-borne viruses, unplanned pregnancy, and physical sexual dysfunction; and which is commonly taken up in research (See Rohleder & Flowers, 2018; Urry, 2020).

The second reason that sexuality is relevant in professional mental healthcare is because sexuality and sexual health are generally theorised through a rights-based perspective, regardless of the specific definition or conceptualisation being utilised. The notion of sexual rights, which refers to the exercise of certain human rights in relation to sexuality and sexual health, has gained wide acceptance in the last two decades (e.g., see Gruskin et al., 2019). From a rights-based perspective, people experiencing any and all forms of mental distress—including those accessing any and all mental health services—are people who retain their fundamental rights related to sexuality, sexual health, and self-expression.

Third, sexuality is relevant in professional mental healthcare because it is an important aspect of person-centred and recovery-oriented care. In many countries including Australia, mental health services are purportedly underpinned by person-centred care and recovery-oriented care principles. Recovery-oriented mental healthcare requires a holistic approach to care that facilitates consumers' self-determination, autonomy, and dignity (Slade et al., 2014). In relation to sexuality, recovery-oriented care requires that the sexuality- and intimacy-related needs or goals that are relevant to and valued by the individual are incorporated

[1] 'Consumer' is the term most used in Australia, akin to the term 'service user' used in some other countries including the United Kingdom. All terms are contentious and it is important to acknowledge that not everyone who experiences distress self-identifies with this term.

into assessment, planning, and care; and consumers are afforded the right to make choices related to sexuality and intimacy that align with their needs and values (Deegan, 1999; also see Urry, 2020).

Sexuality in Mental Healthcare: Current Practice and Research

Research conducted in Australia and internationally consistently reports that sexuality, sexual health, and intimacy are not adequately addressed in professional mental healthcare settings. Evidence demonstrates that mental health clinicians across disciplines and settings continue to be avoidant of sexuality and sexual concerns, or otherwise do not regularly incorporate sexuality-related needs into their regular practice (Berger-Merom et al., 2021; McCann et al., 2019; Higgins et al., 2008; Quinn & Happell, 2015; Quinn et al., 2018; Zatloff et al., 2020). When sexuality-related concerns are addressed in mental health settings, this tends to be in relation to biological dimensions of sexual health or perceived risk and safety concerns (Higgins et al., 2008; Hughes et al., 2018; White et al., 2020). I refer to this broad problem as 'sexuality-related silence', where sexuality and related concerns are ignored, avoided, or reduced to biological and risk-oriented foci. Sexuality-related silence in mental health settings has been widely described but it is still not well understood, evidenced in part by the ongoing nature of the problem despite efforts to intervene and improve sexuality-related practice.

Consistently reported barriers to sexuality-related care across mental health professions include embarrassment or discomfort with the (sensitive) topic—or fear that the consumer will be uncomfortable—and a lack of relevant professional education (e.g., Berger-Merom et al., 2021; McCann et al., 2019; Quinn & Happell, 2015; Quinn et al., 2018; Zatloff et al., 2020). In addition to those barriers, my colleagues and I have demonstrated that clinicians across disciplines and settings may perceive sexuality to be a peripheral issue in mental health settings (Urry et al., 2019). In our study, participating clinicians drew on three explanations (in addition to embarrassment) to account for their own and colleagues' sexuality-related silence. First, that sexuality-related concerns rarely 'come up' in the therapeutic encounter, which was underpinned by an assumption either that consumers do not *have* sexual concerns or that these concerns lack priority for them within the context of their distress. Second, that sexuality is not a priority within the therapeutic encounter compared to other concerns related to an individuals' distress and therapeutic goals, as determined by the clinicians or by the individual themselves. Third, that addressing sexuality-related concerns is not part of mental health clinicians' professional skillsets or roles. The analysis demonstrated how clinicians directly reproduce sexuality-related silence in their accounts by locating sexuality outside of their professional responsibilities and "situating sexuality as peripheral to or not belonging in mental health settings" (Urry et al., 2019, p. 1285).

Available evidence does seem to suggest a clear need to improve clinicians' knowledge, comfort, and competence regarding sexuality-related care. Aligned with this, relevant research commonly advocates for educating and upskilling clinicians as a primary intervention. This approach suggests that sexuality-related silence arises from deficits located *within* clinicians themselves. This positions clinicians as being directly responsible for the problem and it ignores or minimises the role of the broader institution in shaping and constraining clinicians' sexuality-related knowledge, skills, and practice. Given that the problem of sexuality-related silence is ongoing despite increasing research attention over the past 20 years, including the development of interventions aimed at educating and upskilling clinicians directly, it seems that a clinician-focused approach is insufficient to address this problem.

Sexuality-Related Silence: Implicating the Institution

In this section, I argue that when we consider how, why, and when mental health clinicians do not address sexuality, we must also consider the wider context in which those clinicians (and their practice) are embedded. That is, we need to shift the locus of responsibility for sexuality-related silence from clinicians themselves to the broader environment, and institutional context, in which clinicians learn and work (also see Urry et al., 2022).

Institutions can be usefully understood as systems of knowledge that contribute to producing and reinforcing the dominant understandings and practices that provide structure and meaning (Lupton, 2012; McFarland, 2015; Weedon, 1997). They do this within a specific place and time. In the context of mental distress, biomedical or bio-psychiatric discourses are currently dominant in Westernised societies, and these shape understanding of and responses to distress including within professional mental health systems (Sercu & Bracke, 2017). Similarly, biomedical discourses of sexual health, which drive a narrow focus on safety and risk related to biological functions of the sexual body, are currently dominant in healthcare settings within Westernised societies (Ollivier et al., 2019). These and other discourses shape the way that clinicians—healthcare professionals who work within or as part of medical, psychiatric, and psychological institutions—understand and respond to illness experiences and are reproduced through clinicians' professional activities.

The processes through which this occurs can be conceptualised using a theory of professional socialisation, drawn from the work of Emmerich (2015) and Clouder (2003). According to this theoretical perspective, to *become* healthcare professionals, individuals take on the specific cultural or shared knowledge systems belonging to, or constituting, the profession. This inculcation occurs through both informal (or implicit) and formal (explicit) processes; so, for example, both 'hidden curricula' and formal instruction are implicated in the transmission of specific professional values, norms, and modes of thinking (i.e., ways of understanding and responding to illness; Clouder, 2003; Emmerich, 2015). To act and *inter*act meaningfully within their profession, individuals must take up—or challenge—the discourses, norms, and beliefs that are available to them within that professional context (Ollivier et al., 2019). Thus, in becoming and then *being* professionals, individual clinicians draw on and reproduce the profession, or institution, itself.

Importantly, clinicians are not theorised as *passively* reproducing institutional discourses, norms, and beliefs (i.e., they are not 'acted on' by institutional forces; Clouder, 2003; Ollivier et al., 2019): but clinicians' behaviours gain meaning in and through these shared knowledge systems, and so they are *inseparable from* the institution and its broader sociocultural, political, and historical contexts. In relation to sexuality-related silence in mental health settings, that broader context is crucial. As I have argued elsewhere (Urry et al., 2022, p. 545) psychiatry (and related disciplines or professions) has historically "played a central role in defining what is perceived as normative, healthy and acceptable sexuality, sexual expression and relationships" (e.g., Barker et al., 2018; Foucault, 1980; Weeks, 2010). Sexuality was regularly pathologised and regulated, or minimised, in the context of mental distress specifically and there is evidence that this largely continues today, albeit in more subtle forms (See Urry et al., 2022 for a detailed discussion). Certain groups have felt this even more sharply, where mental distress (or perceived mental illness) intersects with gender, race, or diverse sexual identities and behaviours (e.g., see Barker et al., 2018; Grachev et al., 2022; Rees et al., 2021). This wider institutional context and historical silencing of sexuality are important when considering the current and ongoing problem of sexuality-related silence in mental health settings.

Drawing on this theoretical approach, my colleagues and I have demonstrated how sexuality-related silence can be understood as located in the wider institutional context where clinicians learn and work (Urry et al., 2022). Specifically, we demonstrated how this was "*produced* and maintained through institutional processes" situated initially in clinicians' professional education and training and then reinforced through their workplace and professional cultures, and the tools, procedures, and policies that directed their practice (Urry et al., 2022, p. 547; emphasis added). First, clinicians' professional education and training related to sexuality was generally limited, lacking, or absent across all levels. This does not (only) produce a skill deficit, but a particular way of understanding and responding to sexuality within mental health settings. Second, the cultures that many clinicians worked within, both in their local workplace and in their broader professional spheres, were ones in which sexuality was routinely absent or excluded from discussions about mental healthcare planning and provision. Third, and connected to that broader culture of silence, various material and structural constraints (including available tools, policies, and procedures) meant that sexuality was not sufficiently embedded in everyday clinical practice so as to facilitate consistent or affirmative sexuality-related practice. A small and growing body of research has similarly identified or otherwise oriented to the ways in which the wider material, structural, and institutional context shapes clinicians' sexuality-related practice in mental health (e.g., Higgins et al., 2008, 2009; Hughes et al., 2018; White et al., 2020) and other health settings (e.g., Åling et al., 2021). Taken together, this indicates an urgent need to contextualise clinicians' practice and perceptions within that broader institutional context by critically examining those broader workplaces and institutions themselves.

Reframing sexuality-related silence as a problem that is primarily located in the institution itself, rather than in clinicians and their deficits, is useful because it allows us to examine and understand this problem in different ways (Urry et al., 2022). First, this reframing provides an explanation for why we have not yet *solved* the problem through existing approaches and interventions that focus on educating or upskilling clinicians. For example, there are several communication models that aim to support clinicians across a range of health settings to raise and discuss sexuality comfortably (e.g., see Quinn et al., 2012). These models aim to provide a framework for incorporating discussions about sexuality into therapeutic practice, but in doing so, they focus on changing individual clinician's comfort and skills. This remains true even for some models, such as the STARTER model (Luby, 2020), that broadly acknowledge that barriers to discussing sexuality may exist in the clinician's environment rather than the clinician themselves. Moreover, widespread uptake or use of communication models relies on individual clinicians, or clinical managers and supervisors, first identifying a need for improved sexuality-related practice and then taking active steps to achieve this. This is perhaps overly optimistic, given that clinicians may not perceive sexuality to be central or even relevant to their practice (Urry et al., 2019). Locating the problem in the wider institution allows us to consider how communication models and other educational interventions may be useful, but *insufficient alone.*

Second, reframing sexuality-related silence as located primarily in the wider institution provides additional routes or opportunities for change. This reframing implies that any solution to the problem will not be found in (only) trying to 'fix' individual clinicians, but in understanding and shaping an institutional environment, culture, or context that facilitates—or *produces*—improved sexuality-related practice. This is a somewhat daunting task, and one that needs much more attention. To this end, in the next section I outline three broad areas for further critical examination and action: education, service and system cultures, and research.

Moving Forward: Beyond the Clinician's Skills and Deficits

Although I discuss these three areas—education, service and system cultures, and research—separately, they are not intended to be addressed in isolation. Efforts to address any one will necessarily draw on and inform the others. For example, improved professional education and achieving sustained changes to workplace culture will also require—and inform—shifts in research practices.

1. *Professional Education*

There is a clear need to improve formal professional education related to sexuality for mental health clinicians across disciplines, as well the continuing professional education opportunities available to registered clinicians. This is supported by the majority of existing research in this area (e.g., Higgins et al., 2008; Hughes et al., 2018; Quinn & Happell, 2015; White et al., 2020; Zatloff et al., 2020). Importantly, the required 'improvement' is not only about increasing the quantity of sexuality-related training in health professional (students') education. We must also consider, and critically interrogate, *what* is being taught. This is because what is included or excluded in formal curricula constitutes an explicit process of professional socialisation that builds the foundation on which other processes of enculturation occur, for example, during clinical placements, professional specialisation, ongoing experience within the workplace, and through continuing professional education.

What is (and is not) taught within formal pre-registration education provides students with a framework with which to understand and think about sexuality and sexual health within the context of their (future) clinical work. The *absence* of relevant education may indicate to students that sexuality is not relevant in mental health settings and care (Urry et al., 2022). The presence of relevant education that is *narrow* in its scope, for example focusing on biological domains of sexual and reproductive health, provides student clinicians with biomedical, risk-based perspectives with which to navigate sexuality-related needs or concerns within the mental health setting (Higgins et al., 2009; Urry et al., 2022). Certainly, biological domains of sexuality and sexual health are important, but this narrow focus is not well aligned with the WHO's (2006) working definitions; nor does this provide students with an understanding of how sexuality, sexual expression, and intimacy are relevant within the context of mental distress and associated recovery-oriented care. For example, Berger-Merom et al. (2021) reported that mental health clinicians may be ambivalent about the status of sexuality and intimacy-related experiences or issues *as* appropriate recovery-oriented goals. Adequate sexuality-related education must be present *and* comprehensive and affirmative to provide (student) clinicians with a framework to think about, value, and respond to sexuality through rights-based and recovery-oriented perspectives.

Relatedly, there is a need for research that provides a snapshot of the current state of sexuality-related education within schools of nursing, medicine, psychology, and other relevant health professional programmes, both in Australia and globally. Although there is a general agreement within the literature that sexuality-related pre-registration education is not adequate or especially standardised within or across disciplines, it is not clear what *is* being taught or *how varied* such education might be. Understanding what is currently being taught will provide an additional lens through which to consider current sexuality-related practice (or silence), as well as the opportunity to identify any existing examples of good educational practice that can serve as guides for wider curriculum re-development.

2. *Mental Health Services and System Culture*

Locating the problem of sexuality-related silence in the wider institutional context encourages us to focus *on* that broader context as a target of understanding and intervention. Crucially, this also means that efforts to incorporate an affirmative approach to sexuality into mental healthcare must be embedded in workplace cultures and structures because these shape clinicians' practice. Workplace cultures that do not value the inclusion of sexuality in holistic, recovery-oriented care are unlikely to facilitate adequate sexuality-related practice, even if a clinician has the requisite knowledge or skills. Individual clinicians are not necessarily able to practice contra to an existing dominant workplace or professional culture, particularly if they have fewer years' experience or are in a lower hierarchical position (Lupton, 2012). Staff at all levels within a workplace, but particularly clinical managers and supervisors, must value affirmative sexuality-related care. Without this, the relative success of improved pre-registration education would likely be reduced or slowed because the workplaces that junior clinicians enter (or complete clinical placements within) would not facilitate the translation of this acquired knowledge and skill into practice or, more directly, would (continue to) teach the re-production of sexuality-related silence.

Relevant workplace culture change can be facilitated in part through the development or use of tools and guidelines (local or system level) that support current and future clinicians to raise and address sexuality- and intimacy-related concerns within their practice. For example, research involving mental health professionals across a range of disciplines has reported that clinicians themselves identify a need for relevant staff training, guidelines, and tools to indicate the importance and acceptability of—and therefore facilitate improved or more consistent—sexuality-related care within their workplace (e.g., Hughes et al., 2018; White et al., 2020). Researchers should also consider whether tools or their implementation need to be designed differently depending on the type of mental health setting or service, as well as where the service is located and the cultural values and needs of the people involved in the therapeutic encounter.

Overall, there is a need to better understand how clinicians' practice (i.e., their avoidance *and* inclusion of sexuality-related issues) is shaped by their workplaces and workplace culture, and how changes within this context may facilitate, maintain, or constrain changes in practice. More research is needed that examines how sexuality is understood and responded to by the wider workplaces and systems (for an excellent example, see Brown et al., 2014). Importantly, affecting change at the level of workplaces and systems is complex and non-linear (Kitson et al., 2018). This means that we will also need to explore how to best facilitate culture change, including the successful and sustained uptake of specific tools and policies to facilitate sexuality-related practice. The field(s) of implementation of science and knowledge translation may be useful here (e.g., Jull et al., 2017; Kitson et al., 2018). These emphasise the importance of ensuring that interventions are tailored to specific local contexts and led locally by stakeholders (including consumers) rather than simply being 'implemented by' researchers or senior management in a top-down manner. Successful interventions, then, engage clinicians and other stakeholders at all levels within the workplace to achieve a change in the workplace culture itself.

3. *Research*

Research is part of the broader fabric of the institutions that produce sexuality-related silence in mental health settings and the mental health system more broadly. This means that researchers (regardless of whether they are also registered clinicians) are directly implicated in this institutional problem and must contribute to institutional change. We cannot improve educational opportunities, workplace cultures, and material and structural supports if the research underpinning these is itself reproducing narrow or pathologising approaches to sexuality—both broadly (Rohleder & Flowers, 2018) and within the context of mental distress and illness (Urry, 2020). Biological aspects of sexual health continue to dominate research (e.g., Corbett et al., 2017), often despite the explicit use of the WHO's (2006) affirmative and holistic definition of sexual health. These topics are important, but they are not the only aspects of sexuality that are relevant. If we listen to consumers—and we should—these are only some of the sexuality-related concerns or issues that are important and that clinicians should be prepared to discuss, listen to, support, or address (e.g., Deegan, 1999; McCann et al., 2019; White et al., 2021).

Researchers can reflect on how they conduct research in relation to sexuality within the context of mental distress and mental healthcare, for example, by reflexively considering:

- What conceptualisations of sexuality or sexual health they take up *and* how they use or operationalise these within their research.
- The kinds of research questions they ask, as well as the methods of data collection and analysis they select; and how these might limit the kinds of 'answers' they can generate.
- And the use, or potential misuse, of the knowledge they generate and disseminate.

This also includes critically reflecting on how our research, however it is conducted and no matter how well-intentioned, may contribute to further medicalising sexuality by legitimating it as a topic for clinical inquiry and intervention. This issue has been discussed elsewhere (e.g., Mareck & Hare-Mustin, 2009; also see Urry, 2020), but it reinforces the fundamental importance of co-produced and participatory research within this field. Pragmatically, there are many barriers to conducting co-produced research well (Scholz et al., 2019). Researchers seeking to explore sexuality within (mental) health settings should consider seriously how they might take steps to involve various stakeholders, but especially consumers, within their research in meaningful ways.[2] This might be through specific participatory methodologies or other various processes of collaboration or co-production with consumer researchers for example. Even where these approaches are not taken up, research can be better grounded in consumer perspectives by centring the reported experiences and needs of consumers and others who access mental healthcare, as reported in the literature.

[2] I include myself here. To date, my own research has not been co-produced in any meaningful way; I have reflected critically on this (Urry, 2020) and continue to do so.

Conclusion

Sexuality, intimacy, and sexual expression are all potentially important parts of consumers' lives and are therefore relevant within recovery-oriented mental healthcare; yet sexuality-related care in mental health settings globally is largely inadequate. This problem, which I refer to as sexuality-related *silence*, is typically understood as arising directly from individual clinicians' insufficient knowledge, comfort, or competence; and so the solution is sought in addressing these deficits directly. This clinician-focused approach has not achieved effective or sustained change. I have argued for the utility of reframing the problem of sexuality-related silence as one located primarily within the broader institutions where clinicians learn and work. This redirects our focus for both understanding and intervention. Researchers need to work together with clinicians, educators, and consumers to critically examine professional education practices and workplace cultures, as well as reflexively interrogate our own research practices and priorities. We must move forward and make change with care, centring the experiences and needs of consumers and, wherever possible, working *with* and being led by them.

Acknowledgements My sincere thanks to Anna Chur-Hansen, Carole Khaw, and Brett Scholz for their contributions to the research and broader project I have drawn on in this chapter. The original research drawn on in this chapter was supported by a University of Adelaide research scholarship awarded to Kristi Urry by the Faculty of Health and Medical Sciences.

References

Åling, M., Lindgren, A., Löfall, H., & Okenwa-Emegwa, L. (2021). A scoping review to identify barriers and enabling factors for nurse–patient discussions on sexuality and sexual health. *Nursing Reports, 11*(2), 253–266. https://doi.org/10.3390/nursrep11020025

Barker, M. J., Gill, R., & Harvey, L. (2018). *Mediated intimacy: Sex advice in media culture*. Polity Press.

Berger-Merom, R., Zisman-Ilani, Y., Jones, N., & Roe, D. (2021). Addressing sexuality and intimate relations in community mental health services for people with serious mental illness: A qualitative study of mental health practitioners' experiences. *Psychiatric Rehabilitation Journal, 45*(2), 170–175. https://doi.org/10.1037/prj0000506

Burr, V. (2015). Social constructionism (3rd edition). UK: Routledge.

Brown, S. D., Reavey, P., Kanyeredzi, A., & Batty, R. (2014). Transformations of self and sexuality: Psychologically modified experiences in the context of forensic mental health. *Health, 18*(3), 240–260. https://doi.org/10.1177/1363459313497606

Clouder, L. (2003). Becoming professional: Exploring the complexities of professional socialization in health and social care. *Learning in Health and Social Care, 2*(4), 213–222.

Corbett, R., Elsom, S., Sands, N., & Prematunga, R. (2017). An exploratory investigation of sexual health screening in the first 12 weeks of case management in populations with severe mental illness. *International Journal of Mental Health Nursing, 26*(2), 160–169. https://doi.org/10.1111/inm.12257

Deegan, P. E. (1999). Human sexuality and mental illness: Consumer viewpoints and recovery principles. In P. F. Buckley (Ed.), *Sexuality and serious mental illness* (pp. 21–33). Harwood Academic Press.

Emmerich, N. (2015). Bourdieu's collective enterprise of inculcation: The moral socialisation and ethical enculturation of medical students. *British Journal of Sociology of Education, 36*(7), 1054–1072.

Epstein, S., & Mamo, L. (2017). The proliferation of sexual health: Diverse social problems and the legitimation of sexuality. *Social Science & Medicine, 188*, 176–190. https://doi.org/10.1016/j.socscimed.2017.06.033

Foucault, M. (1980). *The history of sexuality* (Vol. 1). Allen Lane.

Grachev, K., Santoro Lamelas, V., Gresle, A. S., de la Torre, L., & Pinazo, M. J. (2022). Feminist contributions on sexual experiences of women with serious mental illness: A literature review. *Archives of Women's Mental Health*, 1–18. https://doi.org/10.1007/s00737-022-01258-0

Gruskin, S., Yadav, V., Castellanos-Usigli, A., Khizanishvili, G., & Kismödi, E. (2019). Sexual health, sexual rights and sexual pleasure: Meaningfully engaging the perfect triangle. *Sexual and Reproductive Health Matters, 27*(1), 29–40. https://doi.org/10.1080/26410397.2019.159378

Higgins, A., Barker, P., & Begley, C. M. (2008). 'Veiling sexualities': A grounded theory of mental health nurses' responses to issues of sexuality. *Journal of Advanced Nursing, 62*(3), 307–317. https://doi.org/10.1111/j.1365-2648.2007.04586.x

Higgins, A., Barker, P., & Begley, C. M. (2009). Sexuality and mental health nursing in Ireland: Weaving the veil of socialised inhibition. *Nurse Education Today, 29*(3), 357–364. https://doi.org/10.1016/j.nedt.2008.07.003

Hughes, E., Edmondson, A. J., Onyekwe, I., Quinn, C., & Nolan, F. (2018). Identifying and addressing sexual health in serious mental illness: Views of mental health staff working in two National Health Service organizations in England. *International Journal of Mental Health Nursing*. https://doi.org/10.1111/inm.12402

Jull, J., Giles, A., & Graham, I. D. (2017). Community-based participatory research and integrated knowledge translation: Advancing the co-creation of knowledge. *Implementation Science, 12*(1), 1–9. https://doi.org/10.1186/s13012-017-0696-3

Kitson, A., Brook, A., Harvey, G., Jordan, Z., Marshall, R., O'Shea, R., & Wilson, D. (2018). Using complexity and network concepts to inform healthcare knowledge translation. *International Journal of Health Policy and Management, 7*(3), 231–243. https://doi.org/10.15171/ijhpm.2017.79

Luby, R. (2020). Using the STARTER model to talk about sex in mental health nursing practice. *Mental Health Practice, 23*(4), 32–41. https://doi.org/10.7748/mhp.2020.e1457

Lupton, D. (2012). *Medicine as culture: Illness, disease and the body*. Sage.

Marecack, J., & Hare-Mustin, R.T. (2009). Clinical psychology: The politics of madness. In D. Fox, I. Prilleltensky, & S. Austin (Eds.), *Critical psychology: An introduction* (2nd ed., pp. 75–92). London: SAGE.

McCann, E., Donohue, G., de Jager, J., Nugter, A., Stewart, J., & Eustace-Cook, J. (2019). Sexuality and intimacy among people with serious mental illness: A systematic review of qualitative research. *JBI Database of Systematic Reviews and Implementation Reports, 17*(1), 74–125. https://doi.org/10.11124/JBISRIR-2017-003824

McFarland, A. S. (2015). Power. In J. D. Wright (Ed.), *International encyclopedia of the social & behavioral sciences* (2nd ed., pp. 760–764). Elsevier.

Murray, M. (2015). Introducing critical health psychology. In M. Murray (Ed.), *Critical health psychology* (pp. 1–16). Palgrave.

Quinn, C., & Happell, B. (2012). Getting BETTER: Breaking the ice and warming to the inclusion of sexuality in mental health nursing care. *International Journal of Mental Health Nursing, 21*(2), 154–162. https://doi.org/10.1111/j.1447-0349.2011.00783.x

Ollivier, R., Aston, M., & Price, S. (2019). Let's talk about sex: A feminist post-structural approach to addressing sexual health in the healthcare setting. *Journal of Clinical Nursing, 28*(3–4), 695–702. https://doi.org/10.1111/jocn.14685

Quinn, C., & Happell, B. (2015). Exploring sexual risks in a forensic mental health hospital: Perspectives from patients and nurses. *Issues in Mental Health Nursing, 36*(9), 669–677. https://doi.org/10.3109/01612840.2015.1033042

Quinn, C., Platania-Phung, C., Bale, C., Happell, B., & Hughes, E. (2018). Understanding the current sexual health service provision for mental health consumers by nurses in mental health settings: Findings from a survey in Australia and England. *International Journal of Mental Health Nursing, 27*(5), 1522–1534. https://doi.org/10.1111/inm.12452

Rees, S. N., Crowe, M., & Harris, S. (2021). The lesbian, gay, bisexual and transgender communities' mental health care needs and experiences of mental health services: An integrative review of qualitative studies. *Journal of Psychiatric and Mental Health Nursing, 28*(4), 578–589. https://doi.org/10.1111/jpm.12720

Rohleder, P., & Flowers, P. (2018). Towards a psychology of sexual health. *Journal of Health Psychology, 23*(2), 143–147. https://doi.org/10.1177/1359105317750162

Scholz, B., Gordon, S., Bocking, J., Liggins, J., Ellis, P., Roper, C., et al. (2019). "There's just no flexibility": How space and time impact mental health consumer research. *International Journal of Mental Health Nursing, 28*(4), 899–908. https://doi.org/10.1111/inm.12589

Sercu, C., & Bracke, P. (2017). Stigma, social structure, and the biomedical framework: Exploring the stigma experiences of inpatient service users in two Belgian psychiatric hospitals. *Qualitative Health Research, 27*(8), 1249–1261. https://doi.org/10.1177/1049732316648112

Slade, M., Amering, M., Farkas, M., Hamilton, B., O'Hagan, M., Panther, G., et al. (2014). Uses and abuses of recovery: Implementing recovery-oriented practices in mental health systems. *World Psychiatry, 13*(1), 12–20. https://doi.org/10.1002/wps.20084

Urry, K. L. (2020). *Sexuality and sexual health in mental health care settings: Perceptions of psychologists, psychiatrists, and mental health nurses in* Australia. Doctoral dissertation.

Urry, K., Chur-Hansen, A., & Khaw, C. (2019). 'It's just a peripheral issue': A qualitative analysis of mental health clinicians' accounts of (not) addressing sexuality in their work. *International Journal of Mental Health Nursing, 28*(6), 1278–1287. https://doi.org/10.1111/inm.12633

Urry, K., Chur-Hansen, A., & Khaw, C. (2022). 'It's not really a part of standard practice': Institutional silencing of sexuality within Australian mental health settings. *Qualitative Health Research, 32*(3), 543–555. https://doi.org/10.1177/10497323211061340

Weedon, C. (1997). *Feminist practice & poststructuralist theory* (2nd ed.). Blackwell Publishers.

Weeks, J. (2010). *Sexuality* (3rd ed.). Routledge.

White, R., Haddock, G., & Varese, F. (2020). Supporting the intimate relationship needs of service users with psychosis: What are the barriers and facilitators? *Journal of Mental Health*, 1–7. https://doi.org/10.1080/09638237.2019.1608928

White, R., Haddock, G., Campodonico, C., Haarmans, M., & Varese, F. (2021). The influence of romantic relationships on mental wellbeing for people who experience psychosis: A systematic review. *Clinical Psychology Review, 86*, 102022. https://doi.org/10.1016/j.cpr.2021.102022

World Health Organization. (2006). *Defining sexual health: Report of a technical consultation on sexual health*, 28–31 January 2002. WHO. https://www.who.int/reproductivehealth/publications/sexual_health/defining_sh/en/. Accessed Dec 2015.

Zatloff, J. P., Silke, A., Philip, Z., & Ward, M. C. (2020). Navigating a complex health system: The perceptions of psychiatric residents in addressing sexual and reproductive health of women with severe mental illness. *Academic Psychiatry*, 1–5. https://doi.org/10.1007/s40596-020-01197-x

12

Romance in the Context of Psychosis: A Risky Business or Are Mental Health Services Just Risk Averse?

Rebecca White, Filippo Varese, Gillian Haddock, and Maria Haarmans

Romantic relationships permeate all areas of our lives, but the romantic relationship needs of mental health service users are often overlooked. This chapter will focus specifically on people who receive a diagnosis of, or have their experiences described as, psychosis and explore how perceptions of risk, in relation to mental health and safety, create a barrier to holistic care. We start with a brief overview of psychosis, its impact on interpersonal relationships, and what recovery might look like. This chapter will then move on to a discussion of risk in relationships and how risk averse attitudes are formed and maintained in mental health services. We discuss the notion of risk regarding romantic relationships in the

R. White (✉) • F. Varese • G. Haddock
University of Manchester, Manchester, UK
e-mail: Rebecca.white@manchester.ac.uk

M. Haarmans
University of Liverpool, Liverpool, UK

Z. Boden-Stuart, M. Larkin (eds.), *Relationships and Mental Health*,
https://doi.org/10.1007/978-3-031-50047-3_12

context of psychosis and conclude by encouraging mental health services to evaluate and reconsider their current attitudes towards the romantic relationship needs of people with experience of psychosis.

Psychosis

'Psychosis' is an umbrella term used to refer to a range of experiences including hallucinations, delusions, disorganised speech, poverty of speech, lack of motivation, as well as an inability to express emotions or experience pleasure (Andreasen, 1982; Arndt et al., 1991; NHS, 2019). Psychotic experiences exist on a continuum of severity, ranging from benign and common to more severe and debilitating. Ongoing and distressing experiences of psychosis may have negative implications on an individual's ability to work, live independently, and maintain social contacts (Joseph et al., 2015). The onset of psychosis is often a catalyst to loss of valued relationships with friends and family, including children and romantic partners (McCarthy-Jones et al., 2013).

Regarding romantic relationships specifically, the experience of psychosis may lead to changes in behaviour which alter the previous dynamic of a relationship (Lewis, 2017). These changes may mean the relationship no longer aligns with a partner's original expectations. For example, they may be required to take on increased caring responsibilities. Some may be accepting of these altered roles, whilst others may not and wish to separate (Lewis, 2017). Additional challenges include the experience of sexual dysfunction as a side effect of antipsychotic medication, difficulties linked to stigma, and poor self-esteem (de Jager et al., 2017; McMillan et al., 2017). Men with psychosis may particularly struggle and are less likely than women with psychosis to have romantic relationships (Firmin et al., 2021; White et al., 2021a). Overall, research suggests there are high levels of loneliness and dissatisfaction with intimate relationships amongst people with psychosis (Badcock et al., 2020; Laxhman et al., 2017). Yet, findings from our research (White et al., 2021b) indicate that romantic relationships are valued and often desired by people with psychosis, as illustrated by the following quote:

I think if I could find somebody like that and grow old with somebody like that that would make me tremendously happy [...] a relationship's what we're all after at the end of the day. (Grant)

There may also be an important role for romantic relationships in recovery from psychosis. Contemporary understandings suggest that recovery is not just about the reduction of symptoms (although for many the reduction of distress surrounding their experiences may be important) but relates closely to the personal goals of individuals. Thus, it places importance on whether a person considers their life to be meaningful and fulfilling (Roe et al., 2011). Measures of 'personal recovery' developed in collaboration with people who have experienced psychosis do not solely assess presence or absence of symptoms; rather, they cover broader items such as 'I feel better about myself', 'I am able to develop positive relationship with other people', and 'I feel that my life has purpose' (Law et al., 2014). Feeling valued by social contacts has been linked to self-esteem and has also been shown to be predictive of subjective recovery in people with psychosis (Frank & Davidson, 2012; Norman et al., 2013). As such, goals around romantic relationships may be an important part of recovery for some.

Although some mental health practitioners may consider it part of their role to provide support around romantic relationships (Southall & Combes, 2020), it is not an area in which mental health services routinely provide support (Hendry et al., 2018; Hughes et al., 2018). This is concerning given that people who experience psychosis may find it challenging to maintain existing relationships or form new ones for the reasons outlined above. Additionally, qualitative research suggests that sexual imagery and experience may be part of the phenomenology of psychosis. For example, voices may threaten sexual violence, be sexualised and derogatory, or include slurs based a person's gender, sexuality, or sexual activity (Haarmans et al., 2016; Jones et al., 2018). Similarly, somatic hallucinations and delusions may be linked to sex, sexuality, or romantic relationships. These experiences might lead to feelings of shame and guilt and therefore be difficult to share with professionals (Jones et al., 2018). However, if not discussed, they could impede recovery.

Risk

There are several reasons why the romantic relationships of people with experience of psychosis are overlooked. Professionals may be concerned about how appropriate it is to discuss romantic relationships with service users. Conversations may be avoided due to the belief they will be embarrassing, uncomfortable, or better left to someone else. Poor access to resources and a lack of training for staff is also a factor (Hendry et al., 2018; Hughes et al., 2018; Southall & Combes, 2020; White et al., 2020). A concept that can be seen as drawing all these issues together is 'risk', specifically, the risk of 'getting it wrong'. A study involving psychologists in England indicated that even professionals who saw conversations about sexuality and romantic relationships as an important part of their job perceived that initiating such conversations could cause a service user to become distressed. Whilst some participants felt that discussions about romantic relationship needs could enhance a therapeutic relationship, others were concerned that such conversations may increase the risk of a client harming themselves or someone else and damage the therapeutic relationship. Those with the latter view stated they would only consider the romantic relationships of service users where there was a related presenting problem and would be unlikely to initiate conversations about relationships otherwise (Southall & Combes, 2020).

Outside of mental health services, a large portion of the general population still endorse stereotypes which conceptualise people with schizophrenia (a diagnosis which includes the experience of psychosis) as dangerous and unpredictable (Wood et al., 2014). These views appear to be present within mental health services when considering the romantic relationships of service users too. A qualitative study found mental health nurses, psychiatrists, and psychologists conceptualised the romantic relationships and sexuality of people with mental health diagnoses as 'dangerous'. Individuals were seen as being dangerous to either themselves or others, with men most often viewed as predatory and a danger to others and women more likely to be seen as vulnerable to abuse, sexually transmitted infections, pregnancy, or sexual disinhibition. As such, healthy romantic relationships are positioned as incompatible with the experience of being mentally unwell (Urry & Chur-Hansen, 2020).

The current authors conducted a qualitative study (White et al., 2020) in which we interviewed professionals from a variety of disciplines working in community mental health services. We aimed to understand the barriers and facilitators regarding the provision of support around romantic relationships. A major theme in our findings related to risk. Mental health professionals described the romantic relationships of people with psychosis as often being turbulent (White et al., 2020). The professionals in our study were concerned about service users' vulnerability to exploitation, but also rejection from romantic partners and the negative impact this may have on a service user's mental health and recovery. In this way risk might be seen as bi-directional and two-fold, with service user and partner both simultaneously potentially vulnerable and dangerous. Ensuring safety and promoting recovery are key aims within mental health services; therefore, relationships were seen as possibly jeopardising or delaying the attainment of these goals.

> *I guess you'd worry about their vulnerability you would worry about the risk of them being maybe exploited in a relationship maybe also capacity [...] you'd maybe worry about if you were encouraging them to seek out relationships that you're maybe putting them at risk of being rejected which might make them feel worse.*

> *[Y]ou could have a worry about somebody who had risk issues so you know people that we work with kind of go in and out of recovery and sometimes can be doing quite well and at other times things are getting really on top of them [...] and the way that they present is very different they can be very angry erm mostly with themselves [...] but sometimes with other people and there can be violence or aggression and I suppose you know there is a worry with some people sort of how are they be able to manage interpersonal relationships.*

Furthermore, mental health professionals feared that if they did provide support around a romantic relationship that transpired to be abusive or resulted in the decline of a service user's mental health, they would be held accountable. Participant accounts revealed a palpable concern about the implications for them professionally if they encouraged relationships that resulted in harm. One participant said:

> *If anything happened with that individual, they're going to be looking at why has that happened? Whose fault was it? If you're the one that's supported them, which has caused that situation to happen, your head will be right on that chopping block.*

Those who have worked in mental health services may be familiar with this sort of worst-case-scenario thinking. These views are also reflected in other research findings. A focus group study indicated competing interests, for 'care', but also 'control' within community services. Practitioners in this study were expected to manage risk and this inhibited their ability to promote social inclusion (Bertram & Stickley, 2005). Additionally, mental health professionals report difficulty implementing practices such as shared decision-making and positive risk-taking within risk averse environments (Holley et al., 2016).

How Are Risk Averse Attitudes Regarding Romantic Relationships Formed and Maintained?

Psycho-social models of psychosis suggest environmental and social factors play a role in the development and maintenance of psychotic experiences (Longdon & Read, 2017). Traumatic events in childhood such as abuse, neglect, and bullying have been shown to significantly increase the risk of psychosis in adulthood (Varese et al., 2012). Therefore, it is likely the people who present to mental health services will have experienced interpersonal trauma. Mental health professionals may be concerned about re-victimisation within current or future relationships. Indeed, there is a large literature which suggests those who have experienced interpersonal violence in childhood often re-experience abuse later in life. For example, a meta-analysis indicated that, on average, just under half of those who experience sexual abuse in childhood will be sexually assaulted again in adulthood (Walker et al., 2019). Similarly, experiencing aggression from romantic partners during adolescence is associated with intimate partner violence in adulthood (Exner-Cortens et al., 2017). Research also suggests that people with mental health difficulties are at increased risk of experiencing violence from a partner compared to the general population (Khalifeh et al., 2015; Trevillion et al., 2012), with women who experience psychosis more likely to be threatened with violence by a partner, family member, or friend and be the victim of physical violence in the home, compared to men with psychosis (van der Stouwe et al., 2021). Additionally, there is evidence which indicates an association between intimate partner violence and psychosis (Boyda et al., 2015; Shah et al., 2018) and, furthermore, stressful life events, such as conflict at home, are associated with relapse for people who have already experienced a first episode of psychosis (Martland et al., 2020). As such, mental health professionals may feel that any romantic relationships embarked upon by people with experience of psychosis, especially women, are more likely to hinder, rather than promote, recovery.

Outside of mental health services, the stigma that surrounds psychosis is related to how people given this diagnosis are portrayed in the media (Bowen et al., 2019). The prominence of biological explanations for psychosis, rather than social causes, is also believed to contribute to ideas about lack of self-control and make it more likely that people with a diagnosis of psychosis will be seen as, in some way, inherently different from the general population (Read et al., 2006). Mental health services operate within this wider context, and it would be idealistic to assume they are impermeable to such attitudes. Clinicians wishing to provide support around romantic relationships may come up against and have to overcome such views and related concerns.

At an organisational level, two key factors create further barriers to the provision of support and may contribute to the maintenance of risk averse attitudes—these are limited time and lack of training or guidance. Firstly, mental health professionals often have large, complex caseloads and limited time. Managing risk is a priority within services and professionals may feel there is insufficient time to focus on and support romantic relationship needs (Urry et al., 2021; White et al., 2020). Initiating conversations with service users about romantic relationships may be seen as creating extra work, especially where input is needed to ensure risk is managed to a level which is deemed acceptable.

> *[Y]ou have to you prioritise, you get a case load you'll immediately go through it and you prioritise the risks and the risk of not having a relationship is well down […] in some ways it's no good this blowing it under the carpet because for them [service users] relationships possibly have been in the past very significant, so it's about how do you work with it, have you got the time? It's ideal world stuff. If you had the resources and the time yes you would do more but frequently you just don't unless they say, 'this is what I want to do' and they prioritise it.*

Secondly, mental health professionals report a lack of training on how to provide support around romantic relationships (Hendry et al., 2018; Hughes et al., 2018; Southall & Combes, 2020; Urry et al., 2021; White et al., 2020). The training that professionals, perhaps particularly mental health nurses and psychiatrists, receive in relation to sexuality and romantic relationships is likely to be from a biological perspective with a focus on risk—i.e., sexual health, sexual dysfunction as a result of medication, and sexual violence (Urry et al., 2021). A lack of training or guidelines may reinforce the idea that mental health services should not provide support around romantic relationships. Although sexual health is mentioned, The UK National Institute for Health and Care Excellence (NICE) guideline for the rehabilitation for adults with complex psychosis does not make reference to romantic relationships specifically (NICE, 2020). This is also true of the clinical guideline for psychosis and schizophrenia in young people (NICE, 2013). Any professionals who do wish to provide support in this area are likely to do so without the safety-net of knowing they have acted according to policy or the reassurance that they have been trained in the necessary skills to support service users with their romantic relationships. This may make the fear of a negative outcome and subsequent repercussions for them personally, as discussed above, even more daunting.

Are Relationships Really that Risky? Potential Benefits of Romantic Relationships

Despite the stereotypes regarding dangerousness, people who experience psychosis are much more likely to harm themselves than others and are also more likely to be victims of violence rather than perpetrators (Appleby et al., 2021; Brekke et al., 2001; de Vries et al., 2018). People who use mental health services are sometimes referred to as vulnerable adults. This term is applied to those deemed unable to protect themselves from exploitation and abuse. Whilst people with psychosis may well have experienced abuse in the past and some may be at risk in the future, to assume that all relationships involving people with psychosis will be negatively experienced is misguided. Interestingly, data from our research (White et al., 2021b) suggest people with psychosis may be simultaneously fearful of exploitation by others *and* demonstrate awareness about how to maintain their personal safety, sometimes describing a retrospective change in behaviour and increased vigilance due to their past experiences. Despite this, some still adopted the language of mental health professionals referring to themselves as 'vulnerable' or a 'vulnerable adult'. In the quote below Michaela talks about the experience of meeting men online. She conceptualises herself as simultaneously 'vulnerable' and 'well clued up'. The experience of finding oneself in a vulnerable situation is one that many will be able to relate to. As many will do, Michaela describes learning from this experience and furthermore describes her ability to protect herself from financial exploitation. Yet, she still characterises herself as 'very vulnerable' despite evidence to the contrary. The use of 'on my own' further suggests the need for others to protect and look after her.

> *[W]ent back to his house and a were trapped. Not doing that again in a hurry [...] very vulnerable on my own [...] never doing that again, I'll never go back to anyone else's house, meet 'em in town next time if I meet anybody. [...] I've had a couple of them ask for money [...] they'll come on like "me mum's ill she's in hospital have you got some money" and I'm like no that's a load of bullshit. Not having any money off me so I know me boundaries, I'm very well clued up me.* (Michaela)

The language used in mental health services constructs people who experience psychosis as vulnerable and in need of protecting despite evidence that this may not always be the case. Where the term 'vulnerable' is applied broadly and accepted without question, there is little room for service users to reclaim autonomy over their safety.

Our research also suggests that professionals may be concerned about the impact that rejection from potential romantic partners might have on the mental health of service users with psychosis (White et al., 2020). In our interviews with people who have experienced psychosis, themes of stigma and discrimination were certainly prominent. Participants discussed how the experience of psychosis left them feeling undesirable to potential partners (White et al., 2021b).

> *[T]here's a lot of prejudice [...] they don't give you a chance if you're mentally ill.* (Jacob)

Indeed, stigma around mental health is prevalent and the experiences of our participants are mirrored in the wider literature. For example, Boysen (2017) found people described as having schizophrenia were rated as less desirable romantic partners than those without a diagnosis by members of the general public (Boysen, 2017).

Regarding relationship breakdown specifically, evidence is lacking. Our recent systematic review on the impact of romantic relationships on the mental wellbeing of people with psychosis found *some* evidence to suggest that being separated from a partner *may* be associated with reduced satisfaction with life, increased suicidality, as well as increased positive and negative symptoms. Interestingly however, there was also evidence to suggest that distress caused by relationship breakdown may be temporary (White et al., 2021a). In the general population, break-ups and the upset they cause may be viewed as 'par for the course' when it comes to romantic relationships. Thus, we should be mindful not to pathologise this experience.

Where the quality of romantic relationships is good, people with psychosis see a partner as a source of company and someone who can provide emotional and practical support (White et al., 2021b). As such, romantic relationships have the potential to promote recovery. Interviews with mental health professionals revealed that they also saw supportive relationships as protective and having the potential to build self-esteem (White et al., 2020).

> *I was talking about self-esteem and worrying about it knocking their self-esteem. At the same time, I really think it would build it as well.*

Similarly, Redmond et al. (2010) found that participants who had experienced psychosis reported that being in a relationship would be seen as a sign of recovery by others and facilitate subjective recovery by increasing confidence (Redmond et al., 2010).

Interestingly, romantic relationships appear to have a bi-directional association with self-esteem. Research with young adults (aged 18–35) from the general population indicates that those who consider themselves to be more attractive and have greater self-confidence in their appearance have higher self-esteem. Importantly, this relationship is partially due to increased self-confidence in regard to romantic relationships (Bale & Archer, 2013). A large longitudinal cohort study found beginning a new relationship was linked to an increase in self-esteem, whilst relationship breakdown was linked to a reduction in self-esteem (Luciano & Orth, 2017). Furthermore, for couples in relationships, self-esteem has also been linked to relationship satisfaction (Erol & Orth, 2017). As such, success and self-confidence regarding romantic relationships is associated with increased self-esteem and higher self-esteem is linked to increased relationship satisfaction. Qualitative research suggests body image and romantic relationships are linked to self-esteem for people with experience of psychosis too (Frank & Davidson, 2012). In clinical populations, the association between romantic relationships and self-esteem may be particularly salient given the known associations between self-esteem and the experience of psychotic symptoms (Barrowclough et al., 2003).

Recommendations

Despite mental health professionals having understandable concerns regarding romantic relationships and psychosis in the context of a risk averse organisational environment, we argue that a more holistic view should be taken. There are several ways in which conversations about romantic relationships may benefit people with experience of psychosis.

Firstly, knowledge about whether the experience of psychosis is related to relationships or sexuality could lead to a more complete understanding of people's difficulties. Equally, desire for a relationship may be a key goal for some. More generally, service users may benefit from discussions and work around how psychosis intersects with their sexuality and romantic relationships. Such conversations may touch on identity, gender, desirability, stigma, and discrimination. Having this information may help improve formulations and ensure service users receive support that is personally meaningful.

Secondly, given the high prevalence of interpersonal trauma in clinical populations, enquiries about current or past relationships would provide space for service users to disclose and receive support for experiences of abuse. Findings from our qualitative study indicated that service users thought it was important that mental health professionals did provide support in situations where relationships were abusive. This included current and historical instances of intimate partner violence (White et al., 2021b). Furthermore, asking about abuse including intimate partner violence is considered best practice in trauma-informed approaches (Sweeney et al., 2016).

Thirdly, the onset of psychosis is likely to impact on previously established relationship dynamics. Although mental health professionals may involve partners in visits and care planning, this is not always the case. When partners are not included it may be even more difficult to understand and cope with what their loved one is experiencing (Wainwright et al., 2015). Therefore, even when service users are in relationships that professionals do not suspect to be abusive, enquiries should still be made as doing so may present opportunities to involve or educate partners. Involving partners and viewing them as more than just 'carers' may increase coping ability and could help prevent the loss of established and valued relationships.

Findings from qualitative studies indicate that *both* mental health professionals and people with psychosis feel a therapeutic alliance needs to be established before conversations about romantic relationships take place (White et al., 2020, 2021b). Research suggests professionals believe service users may have preferences for who they talk to about romantic relationships based on gender or age (White et al., 2020). However, people with experience of psychosis focused more on relational factors, stating a therapeutic relationship could be established where mental health professionals treated them with respect, took an egalitarian approach, and had a genuine, holistic interest in their lives (White et al., 2021b). Therefore, enquires about romantic relationship needs may in fact contribute to the development of a therapeutic alliance. This is important to consider as positive therapeutic relationships with professionals have been linked to hopefulness and social activity (Berry & Greenwood, 2015), both of which are important components regarding personal recovery.

Conclusion

People with experience of psychosis may have goals or needs relating to romantic relationships and benefit from support in this area of their lives. Concerns about risk appear to be at the heart of why the romantic relationship needs of service users with psychosis are currently overlooked by mental health services. We have argued that a more holistic and humane view of relationships should be adopted and that this could lead to improved therapeutic relationships, better recovery outcomes, and increased overall satisfaction in people's lives.

Acknowledgements The authors who like to acknowledge the ESRC who funded the first author's PhD titled 'Exploring Romantic Relationships in the Context of Psychosis: A Mixed Methods Approach'. Thank you also to all participants from the studies cited in this chapter.

References

Andreasen, N. C. (1982). Negative symptoms in schizophrenia: Definition and reliability. *Archives of General Psychiatry, 39*(7), 784–788.

Appleby, L., Kapur, N., Shaw, J., Turnbull, P., Hunt, I., Ibrahim, S., …, Daud, H. (2021). *The national confidential inquiry into suicide and safety in mental health*. Annual Report: England, Northern Ireland, Scotland and Wales.

Arndt, S., Alliger, R. J., & Andreasen, N. C. (1991). The distinction of positive and negative symptoms. *The British Journal of Psychiatry, 158*(3), 317–322.

Badcock, J. C., Adery, L. H., & Park, S. (2020). Loneliness in psychosis: A practical review and critique for clinicians. *Clinical Psychology: Science and Practice, 27*(4), e12345.

Bale, C., & Archer, J. (2013). Self-perceived attractiveness, romantic desirability and self-esteem: A mating sociometer perspective. *Evolutionary Psychology, 11*(1), 147470491301100107.

Barrowclough, C., Tarrier, N., Humphreys, L., Ward, J., Gregg, L., & Andrews, B. (2003). Self-esteem in schizophrenia: Relationships between self-evaluation, family attitudes, and symptomatology. *Journal of Abnormal Psychology, 112*(1), 92.

Berry, C., & Greenwood, K. (2015). Hope-inspiring therapeutic relationships, professional expectations and social inclusion for young people with psychosis. *Schizophrenia Research, 168*(1–2), 153–160. https://doi.org/10.1016/j.schres.2015.07.032

Bertram, G., & Stickley, T. (2005). Mental health nurses, promoters of inclusion or perpetuators of exclusion? *Journal of Psychiatric and Mental Health Nursing, 12*(4), 387–395.

Bowen, M., Kinderman, P., & Cooke, A. (2019). Stigma: A linguistic analysis of the UK red-top tabloids press' representation of schizophrenia. *Perspectives in Public Health, 139*(3), 147–152.

Boyda, D., McFeeters, D., & Shevlin, M. (2015). Intimate partner violence, sexual abuse, and the mediating role of loneliness on psychosis. *Psychosis, 7*(1), 1–13.

Boysen, G. A. (2017). Stigma toward people with mental illness as potential sexual and romantic partners. *Evolutionary Psychological Science, 3*(3), 212–223. https://doi.org/10.1007/s40806-017-0089-5

Brekke, J. S., Prindle, C., Bae, S. W., & Long, J. D. (2001). Risks for individuals with schizophrenia who are living in the community. *Psychiatric Services, 52*(10), 1358–1366.

de Jager, J., Cirakoglu, B., Nugter, A., & van Os, J. (2017). Intimacy and its barriers: A qualitative exploration of intimacy and related struggles among people diagnosed with psychosis. *Psychosis-Psychological Social and Integrative Approaches, 9*(4), 301–309. https://doi.org/10.1080/17522439.2017.1330895

de Vries, B., van Busschbach, J. T., van der Stouwe, E. C. D., Aleman, A., van Dijk, J. J. M., Lysaker, P. H., et al. (2018). Prevalence rate and risk factors of victimization in adult patients with a psychotic disorder: A systematic review and meta-analysis. *Schizophrenia Bulletin, 45*(1), 114–126. https://doi.org/10.1093/schbul/sby020

Erol, R. Y., & Orth, U. (2017). Self-esteem and the quality of romantic relationships. *European Psychologist.*

Exner-Cortens, D., Eckenrode, J., Bunge, J., & Rothman, E. (2017). Revictimization after adolescent dating violence in a matched, national sample of youth. *Journal of Adolescent Health, 60*(2), 176–183.

Firmin, R. L., Zalzala, A. B., Hamm, J. A., Luther, L., & Lysaker, P. H. (2021). How psychosis interrupts the lives of women and men differently: A qualitative comparison. *Psychology and Psychotherapy, 94*(3), 704–720. https://doi.org/10.1111/papt.12317

Frank, D. M., & Davidson, L. (2012). Experiences of self-esteem in outpatients diagnosed with psychosis: A phenomenological study. *Journal of Humanistic Psychology, 52*(3), 304–320.

Haarmans, M., Vass, V., & Bentall, R. P. (2016). Voices' use of gender, race and other social categories to undermine female voice-hearers: Implications for incorporating intersectionality within CBT for psychosis. *Psychosis, 8*(3), 203–213. https://doi.org/10.1080/17522439.2015.1131323

Hendry, A., Snowden, A., & Brown, M. (2018). When holistic care is not holistic enough: The role of sexual health in mental health settings. *Journal of Clinical Nursing, 27*(5–6), 1015–1027.

Holley, J., Chambers, M., & Gillard, S. (2016). The impact of risk management practice upon the implementation of recovery-oriented care in community mental health services: A qualitative investigation. *Journal of Mental Health, 25*(4), 315–322. https://doi.org/10.3109/09638237.2015.1124402

Hughes, E., Edmondson, A. J., Onyekwe, I., Quinn, C., & Nolan, F. (2018). Identifying and addressing sexual health in serious mental illness: Views of mental health staff working in two National Health Service organizations in England. *International Journal of Mental Health Nursing, 27*(3), 966–974.

Jones, N., Rosen, C., Kamens, S., & Shattell, M. (2018). "It was definitely a sexual kind of sensation": Sex, sexual identity, and gender in the phenomenology of psychosis. *Psychosis, 10*(2), 122–131.

Joseph, J., Kremen, W. S., Glatt, S. J., Franz, C. E., Chandler, S. D., Liu, X. H., et al. (2015). Assessment of Lifespan Functioning Attainment (ALFA) scale: A quantitative interview for self-reported current and functional decline in schizophrenia. *Journal of Psychiatric Research, 65*, 102–107. https://doi.org/10.1016/j.jpsychires.2015.04.001

Khalifeh, H., Oram, S., Trevillion, K., Johnson, S., & Howard, L. M. (2015). Recent intimate partner violence among people with chronic mental illness: Findings from a national cross-sectional survey. *The British Journal of Psychiatry, 207*(3), 207–212.

Law, H., Neil, S. T., Dunn, G., & Morrison, A. P. (2014). Psychometric properties of the questionnaire about the process of recovery (QPR). *Schizophrenia Research, 156*(2–3), 184–189.

Laxhman, N., Greenberg, L., & Priebe, S. (2017). Satisfaction with sex life among patients with schizophrenia. *Schizophrenia Research, 190*, 63–67.

Lewis, L. F. (2017). Meta-Ethnography of Qualitative Research on the Experience of Being a Partner to an Individual with Schizophrenia Spectrum Disorder. *Issues in Mental Health Nursing, 38*(3), 219–232. https://doi.org/10.1080/01612840.2016.1259699

Longdon, E., & Read, J. (2017). 'People with problems, not patients with illnesses': Using psychosocial frameworks to reduce the stigma of psychosis. *Israel Journal of Psychiatry and Related Sciences, 54*(1), 24–30.

Luciano, E. C., & Orth, U. (2017). Transitions in romantic relationships and development of self-esteem. *Journal of Personality and Social Psychology, 112*(2), 307.

Martland, N., Martland, R., Cullen, A. E., & Bhattacharyya, S. (2020). Are adult stressful life events associated with psychotic relapse? A systematic review of 23 studies. *Psychological Medicine, 50*(14), 2302–2316.

McCarthy-Jones, S., Marriott, M., Knowles, R., Rowse, G., & Thompson, A. R. (2013). What is psychosis? A meta-synthesis of inductive qualitative studies exploring the experience of psychosis. *Psychosis, 5*(1), 1–16.

McMillan, E., Sanchez, A. A., Bhaduri, A., Pehlivan, N., Monson, K., Badcock, P., et al. (2017). Sexual functioning and experiences in young people affected by mental health disorders. *Psychiatry Research, 253*, 249–255.

NHS. (2019). *Overview – Psychosis*. https://www.nhs.uk/mental-health/conditions/psychosis/overview/

NICE. (2013). *Psychosis and schizophrenia in children and young people: recognition and management*. https://www.nice.org.uk/guidance/cg155/

NICE. (2020). *Rehabilitation for adults with complex psychosis*. https://www.nice.org.uk/guidance/ng181

Norman, R. M. G., Windell, D., Lynch, J., & Manchanda, R. (2013). Correlates of subjective recovery in an early intervention program for psychoses. *Early Intervention in Psychiatry, 7*(3), 278–284.

Read, J., Haslam, N., Sayce, L., & Davies, E. (2006). Prejudice and schizophrenia: A review of the 'mental illness is an illness like any other' approach. *Acta Psychiatrica Scandinavica, 114*(5), 303–318.

Redmond, C., Larkin, M., & Harrop, C. (2010). The personal meaning of romantic relationships for young people with psychosis. *Clinical Child Psychology and Psychiatry, 15*(2), 151–170.

Roe, D., Mashiach-Eizenberg, M., & Lysaker, P. H. (2011). The relation between objective and subjective domains of recovery among persons with schizophrenia-related disorders. *Schizophrenia Research, 131*(1–3), 133–138.

Shah, R., Von Mach, T., Fedina, L., Link, B., & DeVylder, J. (2018). Intimate partner violence and psychotic experiences in four U.S. cities. *Schizophrenia Research, 195*, 506–512.

Southall, D. J. L., & Combes, H. A. (2020). Clinical psychologists' views about talking to people with psychosis about sexuality and intimacy: A Q-methodological study. *Sexual and Relationship Therapy*, 1–25.

Sweeney, A., Clement, S., Filson, B., & Kennedy, A. (2016). Trauma-informed mental healthcare in the UK: What is it and how can we further its development? *Mental Health Review Journal, 21*, 174.

Trevillion, K., Oram, S., Feder, G., & Howard, L. M. (2012). Experiences of domestic violence and mental disorders: A systematic review and meta-analysis. *PLoS One, 7*(12), e51740. https://doi.org/10.1371/journal.pone.0051740

Urry, K., & Chur-Hansen, A. (2020). Who decides when people can have sex? Australian mental health clinicians' perceptions of sexuality and autonomy. *Journal of Health Psychology, 25*(13–14), 2188–2199. https://doi.org/10.1177/1359105318790026

Urry, K., Chur-Hansen, A., & Khaw, C. (2021). 'It's not really a part of standard practice': Institutional silencing of sexuality within Australian mental health settings. *Qualitative Health Research*, 10497323211061340.

van der Stouwe, E., Steenhuis, L., Pijnenborg, G., de Vries, B., Bartels-Velthuis, A., Castelein, S., et al. (2021). Gender differences in characteristics of violent and sexual victimization in patients with psychosis: A cross-sectional study. *BMC Psychiatry, 21*(1), 1–9.

Varese, F., Smeets, F., Drukker, M., Lieverse, R., Lataster, T., Viechtbauer, W., et al. (2012). Childhood adversities increase the risk of psychosis: A meta-analysis of patient-control, prospective-and cross-sectional cohort studies. *Schizophrenia Bulletin, 38*(4), 661–671.

Wainwright, L. D., Glentworth, D., Haddock, G., Bentley, R., & Lobban, F. (2015). What do relatives experience when supporting someone in early psychosis? *Psychology and Psychotherapy: Theory, Research and Practice, 88*(1), 105–119.

Walker, H. E., Freud, J. S., Ellis, R. A., Fraine, S. M., & Wilson, L. C. (2019). The prevalence of sexual revictimization: A meta-analytic review. *Trauma, Violence, & Abuse, 20*(1), 67–80.

White, R., Haddock, G., & Varese, F. (2020). Supporting the intimate relationship needs of service users with psychosis: What are the barriers and facilitators? *Journal of Mental Health, 29*(3), 314–320. https://doi.org/10.1080/09638237.2019.1608928

White, R., Haddock, G., Campodonico, C., Haarmans, M., & Varese, F. (2021a). The influence of romantic relationships on mental wellbeing for people who experience psychosis: A systematic review. *Clinical Psychology Review, 86*, 102022. https://doi.org/10.1016/j.cpr.2021.102022

White, R., Haddock, G., Varese, F., & Haarmans, M. (2021b). "Sex isn't everything": Views of people with experience of psychosis on intimate relationships and implications for mental health services. *BMC Psychiatry, 21*(1), 307. https://doi.org/10.1186/s12888-021-03262-7

Wood, L., Birtel, M., Alsawy, S., Pyle, M., & Morrison, A. (2014). Public perceptions of stigma towards people with schizophrenia, depression, and anxiety. *Psychiatry Research, 220*(1), 604–608. https://doi.org/10.1016/j.psychres.2014.07.012

13

"You Don't Even Get a Hug": Sexuality and Relational Security in Secure Mental Healthcare

James P. Ravenhill, Paula Reavey, Steven D. Brown, and Zoë Boden-Stuart

Sexuality—including positive relational experiences with self and others—underpins mental health, contributes to recovery from distress, and contributes to "the totality of being a person" (McCann, 2000, p. 134). As such, sexuality is an important dimension of what Stern (2010) and Fuchs (2013) refer to as vitality, or the feeling of being alive. In secure

J. P. Ravenhill (✉)
Royal Holloway, London, UK
e-mail: james.ravenhill@rhul.ac.uk;

P. Reavey
London South Bank University, London, UK

S. D. Brown
Nottingham Business School, Nottingham Trent University, Nottingham, UK

Z. Boden-Stuart
The Open University, Milton Keynes, UK

Z. Boden-Stuart, M. Larkin (eds.), *Relationships and Mental Health*,
https://doi.org/10.1007/978-3-031-50047-3_13

mental healthcare[1] settings, some patients[2] report experiencing the wards as "anti-life", spaces where meaning is obscured. In such spaces, sexualities exist in an "amputated" state, suspended in a liminal space until they may be re-embraced in the outside world (Brown et al., 2014). These spaces are environments of prohibition, where intimate and sexual relationality, including sexual feelings and behaviours, becomes recoded as "misbehaviour" (Ravenhill et al., 2020). The chapter that follows first addresses the "outside-in", introducing the concept of relational security and focusing on current practice ("the external"); it then provides an "inside-out" account of two forensic mental health patients' experiences with sexuality ("the internal"), in order to argue for the need for policy and guidelines to support the well-being and recovery of these patients.

Outside-In: Relational security

Secure mental healthcare services in England are differentiated from general adult services on various factors. Unlike the latter, they are exclusively single-gender and offer "halls of residence"-style accommodation, with access to leisure facilities, creative pursuits, and green spaces. They are also stratified according to the level of risk patients are believed to pose to themselves (low secure) and others (medium and high secure; NHS, 2022). Other mental health services, such as acute psychiatric wards, may have secure conditions in place, but whereas these provide short-term accommodation of up to 30 days, patients residing in secure services tend to stay for prolonged periods, with up to a fifth of those in medium secure and quarter of those in high secure services, spending at least a decade in continuous detainment (Hare Duke et al., 2018). People residing in secure services are often referred to as "forensic" patients, either because they have a history of offending and are under a criminal justice

[1] Secure mental healthcare services (also "secure services" and "forensic services") in England provide accommodation and treatment to people experiencing mental distress, who require the provision of security. Patients may enter directly from prison, or from hospitals, sometimes following arrest.

[2] We use the term "patient", as opposed to service-user, to acknowledge the involuntary nature of detention.

section or because they are believed to pose too great a risk of harm to be cared for in general mental healthcare. It follows that on these wards, concerns regarding care and security are inevitably, inextricably connected.

"Security" in secure mental healthcare is comprised of three elements: physical (or environmental, including the design of buildings, estates, and observation systems), procedural (e.g., the monitoring of patients' movements and communications; risk management and contingency planning), and relational. The latter can be conceptualised in quantitative terms—for example, staff-patient ratio—but also encompasses qualitative aspects, such as the nature of relationships between patients and the care team (Kennedy, 2002; Tighe & Gudjonsson, 2012). These three elements are not mutually exclusive: for example, the physical design of the ward can determine the potential for and quality of in-person contact (see Reavey et al., 2017). All three contribute to ward "safety" and to therapeutic outcomes for patients. However, it is relational security that is arguably the most important for maintaining patients' therapeutic progress and contributing to recovery (Kennedy, 2002). Despite this, when compared to the attention paid in policy, training, research, and ward practice to physical and procedural security, relational security has historically been "the poor relation" (Tighe & Gudjonsson, 2012, p. 185). There has been a great deal of attention paid to physical and procedural security, in policy, training, research, and ward practice, but in comparison, relational security has been under-considered. This is likely owing to a lack of clarity surrounding how relational security should be defined and measured (Chester et al., 2017). Whilst the quantitative aspects of relational security, often conceptualised via their connection to physical and procedural security, have been operationalised in terms of contact times, staff turnover, staff-patient ratios, etc., the qualitative aspects—including the nomenclature of "boundaries" and "purposeful" and "therapeutic" relationships—are less well defined and therefore harder to measure (Chester et al., 2017; Chester & Morgan, 2012; Tighe & Gudjonsson, 2012).

Though not synonymous, social climate and relational security are theoretically similar constructs. "Social climate" encompasses the physical conditions of mental healthcare wards and the social relationships that play out within them (Doyle et al., 2017). Relational security might be conceptualised as an *outcome* of the social climate within the ward. Academic interest in psychiatric "ward milieu" dates back to Caudill's ethnographic work in the 1950s (Caudill, 1958) but became formalised with Moos' studies into the differential effects of ward environments on the behaviour of patients and staff, and a growing understanding that the "social atmosphere" of psychiatric wards was likely to influence therapeutic outcomes (Moos, 1967). Moos' observations inspired him to develop the first measure of social atmosphere, the Ward Atmosphere Scale (WAS), that measured relationship dimensions and personal growth opportunities (which map onto relational security) and system maintenance dimensions (which speak to physical and procedural security; Moos & Houts, 1968).

Moos' work is credited with stimulating empirical enquiry into what is now more commonly referred to as "social climate" and for providing a tool to measure previously unoperationalised concepts, although it has not been without critique (Alden, 1978; Schalast et al., 2008; Tonkin, 2016). Concerns also exist regarding the relevance of the WAS for the twenty-first century: the original authors report reading *One Flew over the Cuckoo's Nest* to inspire the development of scale items. More recently, Schalast et al. (2008) developed the Essen Climate Evaluation Schema (EssenCES), a measure of psychiatric ward social climate that has received consistent empirical support (Tonkin, 2016). The EssenCES encompasses three factors: therapeutic hold (e.g., "Staff take a personal interest in patient progress"); patients' cohesion and mutual support (e.g., "The patients care for each other"); and safety (e.g., "Some patients are afraid of other patients"). However, the EssenCES was not developed to measure relational security per se, and the scale does not contain items relating to how staff use the information they have about patients or how decisions concerning patients are made, so it cannot reliably be used to operationalise this complex construct (Tighe & Gudjonsson, 2012).

Relational Security in Forensic Mental Healthcare

Official guidance for staff working in UK forensic mental healthcare, first published in the Royal College of Psychiatrists-commissioned handbook *See, Think, Act* (STA), describes relational security as "the knowledge and understanding we have of a patient and of the environment, and the translation of that information into appropriate responses and care" (Allen, 2015, p. 5). Written for all staff, from clinicians to administrators to domestic staff, and developed in response to a number of "near-miss" security incidents, *See, Think, Act* (STA) comprises four domains: Inside world, Outside world, Team, and Other patients (Allen, 2015; Tighe & Gudjonsson, 2012). Elements in the "Inside world" domain emphasise the importance of knowing patients' unique histories and "trigger points" and ensuring that the physical environment is conducive to positive social interactions. The "Outside world" domain is concerned with the management of visitors and the monitoring of patients' interactions with people outside of the healthcare service. The "Team" domain centres on the importance of establishing clear boundaries and providing purposeful therapy. "Other patients" focuses on the implications of the dynamic produced by the mix of patients on the ward and the need for staff to monitor how patients interact with each other (Allen, 2015). Therefore, relational security as conceptualised by the Department of Health/Royal College of Psychiatrists provides a potential conceptual framework for developing policies to manage patients' relationships both within and outside services.

The STA guidance and the related tool, the *Relational Security Explorer* (RSE: Royal College of Psychiatrists, 2022), emphasise *staff knowing patients' individual circumstances and histories*, echoing the "personalisation" agenda set out in the National Health Service (NHS) England's (2016) *Five-Year Forward View for Mental Health*, which also advocates the importance of healthy and stable relationships for recovery. However, the heavy emphasis on the therapeutic benefits of positive *staff-patient* relationships in the STA guidance is inversely mirrored by the jarring absence of any mention of the potential for patients to form (potentially therapeutic) romantic or emotionally and/or physically intimate relationships *with each other* and/or to maintain similar, existing connections with people outside. The STA guidance directs staff to be "alert to the possibility of inappropriate attachments to other patients" (Allen, 2015, p. 25), and although it does acknowledge that connections with family and friends should be encouraged, there is no advice as to how staff might navigate patients' *existing* romantic relationships. Formal guidance and policies to guide clinicians' management of such relationships do not appear to be forthcoming: The Royal College of Psychiatrists' (2017, p. 11) report on sexual boundaries in secure mental healthcare acknowledges patients' rights to pursue romantic relationships during detainment, while noting that "[clinicians'] interference" may be warranted for the "protection of [inpatients'] health". Consequently, individual clinicians, or more often other ward staff, are left to decide whether patients' intimate/romantic relationships should be facilitated or obstructed, without any formal guidance as to how such decisions might be reached. Confronted with the reality of intimate and sexual relationships forming between patients, some of whom will be detained for many years, mental healthcare providers typically delegate responsibility to individuals—often the least trained, most precariously employed. This leads to the implementation of inconsistent and ad-hoc ward-based practices, typically centred on prohibition (Dein et al. 2016; Ravenhill et al., 2020).

Secure mental healthcare providers' prohibitive approaches to patients' emotionally and physically intimate relationships are often justified within discourses of vulnerability and risk, wherein patients' desire for intimacy is constructed as discordant with treatment goals, symptomatic of mental distress, and likely to lead to more harm than good (Bartlett et al., 2010; Brown et al., 2014; Hunter & Ahmed, 2016; Ravenhill et al., 2020; Ruane & Hayter, 2008). Staff members' beliefs that people in forensic mental healthcare should have the agency to initiate and/or maintain intimate and sexual relationships may conflict with beliefs regarding the patients' rights to such freedom, given their offending history (Dein et al., 2016; Ruane & Hayter, 2008). Other concerns held by staff include: doubts about patients' capacity to consent to sexual activity; risk of sexual exploitation, abuse and violence; the potential for accusations of rape or abuse; the possibility of condomless sex increasing the risk of sexually transmitted infections and HIV transmission; pregnancy; and the possibility of transactional sex (Dein et al., 2007; Dein & Williams, 2008; Hunter & Ahmed, 2016; Quinn & Happell, 2016; Series, 2014). In the absence of clear policies, ward staff tend to be, understandably, risk-averse in the way they approach patient sexuality and are more likely to interpret intimate relationality—including sexual activity—as instances of "organisational misbehaviour", or deliberate rule-breaking, rather than as attempts by patients to nourish an important aspect of their personhood (Ravenhill et al., 2020).

Given that detention in secure forensic mental healthcare services arises in part because the person is deemed unsafe to themselves and/or others, it is perhaps not unreasonable that security underpins discussions over the freedoms that patients should be able to access. For staff working in forensic mental healthcare, the prohibition of intimate connections between patients—and the monitoring of "inappropriate attachments"—is fundamental to maintaining relational security. However, this overwhelming focus on risk management (Jacob & Holmes, 2011), and in particular the heavy emphasis on physical safety (Curtis et al., 2013), has obscured discussion around the potential benefits to relational security of supporting and facilitating intimate and sexual patient relationships where they are wanted and/or occurring. An illustrative example comes from efforts made by the UK's Care Quality Commission (2018) to address the sexual safety of patients in secure mental healthcare, which focus almost exclusively on issues of consent and predatory behaviour. Although patently extremely important considerations, and part of the healthcare providers' duty of care, sole focus on them obscures broader interpretations of sexual safety, such as managing emotionality and navigating "feeling sexual".

Relational Security and Recovery

Providing support for personal recovery from mental ill-health has become one of the key goals for mental health services in England and Wales (NHS, 2016). Though its meaning remains contested, Shepherd et al. (2008) describe recovery as an individual's right to a meaningful, hopeful, and purposeful life, irrespective of the ongoing presence of "symptoms" of poor mental health. With their emphasis on managing risk, forensic services face significant challenges in honouring a commitment to a recovery-focused approach. Drennan and Alden (2012) suggest that it is necessary to distinguish between recovery in general mental healthcare and recovery in forensic services specifically. "Secure recovery" acknowledges that offending behaviour can arise from mental and emotional distress, emphasises the need to manage risk as part of recovery, and embraces the principle of working towards the restoration of a meaningful *and safe* life (Drennan & Alden, 2012). Concepts like relational security provide a basis for advocating a *therapeutic* understanding of "security" (Kennedy, 2002) and are therefore, theoretically, aligned with a recovery-focused approach. Indeed, forensic patients identify positive relationships with staff, based on feeling respected, valued, and cared for (the cornerstones of the STA guidance), as crucial for facilitating recovery (Clarke et al., 2016). Experiencing these positive staff-patient relationships supports patients' self-esteem and facilitates self-discovery, by enabling a recoding of relational expectations that, owing to adverse life experiences, were often built around feelings of loss, rejection, and mistrust (Clarke et al., 2016; Laithwaite & Gumley, 2007). The construction of a "new and improved" sense of self is one of the three overarching changes that forensic patients report as being constitutive of "recovery", along with making sense of the past and understanding the role of mental ill-health in their lives. Developing a positive relationship *with the self* is a key aspect of recovery (Shepherd et al., 2016).

It is perhaps unsurprising that relationships with staff are of such significance to forensic patients, given how few opportunities they have to develop and maintain relationships with other patients (openly at least), and even fewer with people outside of the service. However, notably lacking from the literature on forensic patients' perspectives on recovery is any mention of the role of positive *intimate* and/or *sexual* relationships. It is important that this is addressed, given the importance of sexuality to embodied self-hood, the risks associated with sexuality existing in an "amputated" or "liminal" state during periods of detainment, and the long-term implications of such for meaningful, "successful" relationality following community discharge (Brown et al., 2014; Reavey et al., 2022).

Inside-Out: Patient Experiences of Intimate and Sexual Relationality in Forensic Mental Healthcare

In this section, we present the experiences of 2 of the 29 patients we interviewed in our research on intimate and sexual relationality in forensic mental healthcare facilities and stepdown services in England (*Feeling sexual inside and out*). This project is part of a programme of research privileging patients' experiences of feeling and being sexual, and staff members' experiences of their patients' relationality and sexuality, which aims to inform the development of policies for people working in secure mental healthcare, so that intimate and sexual relationships, and the centrality of sexuality to personhood, are not overlooked in discussions of relational security or personal recovery. This project took place in a number of medium and low secure and "locked" facilities[3] and in housing services oriented to providing scaffolded transition from secure care to unsupervised community living.

None of the mental healthcare services wherein we undertook research had established policies around managing patient intimate and sexual relationality. The research required the team to navigate pervasive concerns regarding risk, vulnerability, and the "appropriateness" of engaging patients and staff in forensic mental healthcare in conversations about sexuality and intimate relationships.

Our research was informed by contemporary phenomenological theory, in particular Stern's (2010) and Fuchs' (2013) writings on vitality. Vitality describes how alive or well we feel at any moment. It is shaped by the circumstances of our existence and describes our "background" experience in relation to the world and others. In order to gather phenomenological descriptions of what it *feels like* to be a sexual being while living in secure care, we employed a multi-modal data collection approach, combining semi-structured interviews with a drawing methodology (Boden & Eatough, 2014; Reavey & Brown, 2021). At various points during the interviews, participants were asked to draw anything, either literal or

[3] Locked facilities, which provided in-hospital step-down services to prepare patients for community discharge, were retired in October 2021.

abstract, that captured their feelings and experiences of being sexual—a concept that they were encouraged to interpret freely and broadly. Though the drawings made by participants were not treated as data per se, employing the multi-modal approach was intended to facilitate richer verbal responses relating to relationships, sexuality, and mental health and to help participants articulate aspects of embodied experience that might otherwise be difficult to verbalise. Interview questions encouraged participants to use imagery and metaphor to help them convey their embodied feelings. To supplement the verbal data, we recorded in research diaries our observations of various aspects of the interview, including impressions of the ward environment, information provided to us informally by staff, interactions between those living and working on the wards, and participants' nonverbal behaviour during interviews. From these data, we produced richly descriptive profiles for each participant, charting experiences both within and outside secure care, and their embodied experiences of intimate and sexual relationality while detained on the wards. We present two of these participant profiles here.

The participant profiles selected illustrate the potential implications of a failure to attend to the intimate and sexual aspects of patients' relationalities while they are under treatment in forensic mental healthcare. Both patients were residents in the same mental healthcare facility in England at the point of data collection, though living in different wards. Both provided detailed accounts of their experiences of feeling and being sexual and of the consequences of the service's failure to adequately support this area of their experience for their day-to-day lives, their long-term relational goals, and their mental health and recovery. The participants we present here—"Brianna", a 34-year-old woman, and "Jake", a 21-year-old man—were selected because their unique experiences reflect a range of potential consequences of overlooking intimate and sexual relationality for a *therapeutic interpretation* of relational security—and for patient care.

Brianna

Brianna is staying in a low secure ward for treatment and recovery, having received a diagnosis of a personality disorder. She is from the Caribbean, but moved to the UK when she was 19. Brianna has been at the current hospital for four-and-a-half years and was previously in prison. Brianna hears voices and is particularly acquainted with one of them, hip-hop singer Trevian [name changed], who makes highly sexualised music videos featuring women who "twerk".

Brianna is nostalgic about her time in the Caribbean, missing the days when she would "go to the dancehall, dancing with her friends… dancing with guys". The dances would be "exotic", "sexual", and "outrageous" and involved "winding and twerking". Now, Brianna "dance[s] every night in [her] room": She "put[s] lingerie on, and stockings, and she just stand[s] around and dance[s] in there on [her] own", the same dances [she] would dance in the dancehall. The voices "like it when [she] does that". Trevian (who is the good voice; there are also bad voices) is "in [her] room" when she dances, and "he likes it when [she] dances around, and put[s] on heels". Brianna believes that "Trevian is a guy who fancies [her]" and "wants [her] to be his girl". According to Brianna, Trevian stands in her room "by the bathroom door, and he's never going to go away. And he's there night and day." Trevian "sticks up" for Brianna, helping to "get rid of the negative voices" who are "bullying" and "controlling". Brianna "loves Trevian, and will do anything to please him". The dancing "makes [her] feel like… [she's] active, [she's] actually doing something…. It keeps [her] occupied, it keeps [her] motivated, and it just makes [her] feel a lot better to do the little dance for a little while." She hasn't told anyone else about her dancing, because that "type of dancing is not exactly what [the staff] would have expected". Brianna told the interviewer that he was the first person to whom she had related the details of her nightly dancing routine and enjoyed sharing the information, because she was "bringing herself out to a stranger".

Trevian "used to give Brianna a lot of orgasm[s]", "but since of lately it's not happening to her anymore". Brianna isn't sure why, but it could be that Trevian "didn't want [her] to do it [have orgasms] in the first place". Brianna has told her Care Co-ordinator that Trevian no longer gives her orgasms, but she "didn't tell her how [she] feels" about it—she "didn't tell her that [she] actually misses it".

Brianna thinks about her sexuality "all the time". When in "the lonely mood", she uses a vibrator, but this "has to be agreed in ward round before [she] can have it". She "wish[es] that [she] could really do something, make love to somebody, kiss. [She] miss[es] kissing somebody." That said, not being sexually active "makes [her] feel good about [her]self" and makes her "feel clean". She has come "into thinking that maybe it's for the best". Brianna believes that patient sexuality "doesn't really matter to staff", and when it comes to patients being inactive sexually, "they look at that as something good": Staff "think that [patients] deserve it, they deserve to not have a relationship, not to be sexually active".

Brianna had found her own unique way of being sexual in the private space she inhabited on the ward, through erotic dancing intended for the man (albeit not an embodied being) with whom she experienced a close sexual relationship. Dancing contributed to Brianna's positive mental health—it made her feel "active" and connected to the man she loved—and yet she had not shared her nightly routine with the healthcare workers charged with facilitating her recovery, uncertain as to how they would respond: The ward was not a place for dancing "like a stripper", notwithstanding its potential therapeutic value. In accordance with the *See, Think, Act* guidance, Brianna's Care Co-ordinator knew the *factual* elements of her "inside world", including her voice-hearing experiences, and even the sexual experiences her voices afforded, but did not know what it *felt like* to Brianna to have these experiences. If recovery can be conceptualised as inclusive of continued symptomology (Shepherd et al., 2008), then Brianna's dancing might be facilitative of her recovery, but in a context where expressions of sexuality are framed as inappropriate (Allen, 2015), recoded as "misbehaviour" (Ravenhill et al., 2020), and interpreted in terms of symptomology (Brown et al., 2014), there is no opportunity for staff to explore the implications of these practices for the long-term well-being of the patient.

In the course of her interview, Brianna intimated a history of sexual exploitation by men, though (because care records were not accessed as part of our research) it is unknown whether this information was known by ward staff. Even if it were not, clinicians would no doubt have concerns over the extent to which Brianna's clandestine nocturnal dance routines—enacted to please an audience of men, who had the power to govern her sexual pleasure—facilitated her recovery or rather evidenced (and contributed to) sustained distress. However, with staff seemingly entirely unaware of her nocturnal pursuits, these concerns neither had the space to be realised nor were addressed, and their potential to enable or constrain some sort of growth for Brianna remains unknown (Reavey et al., 2022).

Jake

Jake is staying in a medium secure ward offering assessment and rehabilitation to young adults. He has been in secure services since he was 13 years old, having committed a criminal offence. Jake is currently in a relationship with a considerably older man, who is not a patient.

Jake entered secure services at a point where he was confused over his sexual orientation and did not have a reliable source of information about issues related to sexuality. Jake was prohibited from talking about his index offence when he was first in hospital, and he generalised this imposed silence to other issues of concern. Consequently, sexuality "became an extra thing [he] couldn't talk about that was on [his] mind". Jake had difficulties "becoming comfortable with being gay" and "how [he] could express that". Hospital staff were not wholly supportive of Jake's desire to explore his sexual identity: "Some of the staff, bullied [him] a bit, and some of the bank staff said it was God testing [him]."

At one point, Jake had a "little bit of an encounter" with another patient, and staff "were really funny over it, and [he] got told how far it had set [him] back". When Jake was able to take unescorted leave, "the first thing [he] wanted to do was to go on Grindr", something he really had to "argue for". Staff were not supportive of Jake's request to use Grindr: They told him that he was "delaying himself getting out", that his "priorities are all wrong", and that he "should not be thinking about relationships until he was discharged". Jake was undeterred: He wanted to experience "all of it, every little detail of it. [He] wanted to set up a profile, have people messaging him, and the thrill of it all, and end up meeting up with someone, and then go back to theirs." When he was allowed to download Grindr, he "met someone and went back to theirs, and the staff told [him] [he]'d broken Section 17 of his leave, and they took [his] leave off [him]." Jake was "always told that patients could be honest with staff, but [he] had a lot of staff telling [him], 'Don't tell [clinicians], just do whatever you want to do, just don't get caught doing it.'" It ended up that Jake "started meeting up with people and going back and just not telling staff [he]'d done it when [he] got home".

Jake's psychologist told him that if he were to meet up with someone he had met on Grindr, they should meet in a public place. On reflection, he thinks the psychologist must have meant somewhere like a hotel, but at the time, Jake thought that "the toilets of [a large exhibition centre] sounded fine". Once again, when he was "honest" with the staff about the encounter, he was sanctioned with loss of leave. Jake thought that "by doing it there [he] wouldn't be in trouble with [his] leave plan" because it was a public place. Jake now refers to this incident as his "Dorian Green moment" (*Dorian Green is a character from the British television show* Birds of a Feather, *who is renowned for being promiscuous*). To Jake, meeting people for sex was worth the risk of losing benefits, because doing so "made [him] feel so complete and wanted, and everything [he] was missing in [his] life, it made [him] feel like he had. Not even the sex side of it, just the intimacy." It was "an amazing feeling" to be "cuddled up, entwined with someone, safe and secure", when "in hospital, you didn't even get a hug off anyone" and where "everything feels cold". Jake sees his "sexuality and self-worth and mental health being entwined".

Jake's relationship with his current partner—whom he met via Grindr—has not run smoothly. Once, Jake lost his leave because his partner "talked about breaking up because he couldn't cope with it all" and, in response, Jake "came up with the plan of running off to [Spain]", a plan which Jake "ended up roping his partner into", and that was eventually realised. He did it "knowing [he] was going to get caught, because [he] wanted to prove to [his] partner how much [he] loved him". When he was apprehended, Jake ended up in prison.

Jake had learned that sharing information about his sexual relationships with his care team was a mistake, because it resulted in punishment.

A culture of silence around sexuality—along with homophobic attitudes among some staff—meant that Jake was forced to explore his sexual identity without many of the structures that would otherwise have supported his identity formation as a gay man. Reasonable expectations that the "freedom" afforded by unescorted leave might enable him to explore sexual relationships were shattered by staff members' recoding of his sexual desires as something that would detract, and distract focus, from his recovery. The temporal logics of recovery mean that focusing on "getting better" precedes any investment in intimate and sexual relationality: Infractions are not only "misbehaviour", but they are evidence of a failure in recovery. Patients are therefore obliged to navigate the tensions between the freedoms of the outside world—which can feel full of sexual possibilities—and the prohibitive, oppressive restrictions of the ward, where sexual feelings have to be "turned off" and never spoken of.

It is perhaps understandable that ward staff and clinicians were keen to constrain Jake's keen sexual motivations, concerned that emotional and sexual immaturity could make him vulnerable to other men on the ward and expose other patients to risk, especially in light of his earlier "encounter" with a wardmate. However, in Jake's case, a strong desire to explore his sexuality, his longing for romantic intimacy, his knowledge of the availability of sex and intimacy in the outside world, and his understanding that "keeping quiet" about these things was the most effective way of avoiding punishment, were a recipe for disaster. In the absence of a safe forum to help him manage his sexual feelings, Jake resorted to absconding and was subsequently arrested—a substantial failure in relational security. Paradoxically—though not surprisingly—attempts at maintaining relational security via supposedly risk-diminishing practices (restriction and prohibition) actually *increase* the risk to ward and patient safety and can have serious consequences for recovery.

Intimacy and Sexuality in Relational Security

The experiences described by Brianna and Jake (the "inside-out") highlight the threats to relational security, in particular to the well-being and recovery of patients, that arise as a consequence of failures to account for intimate and sexual relationality in secure mental healthcare policy and local staff guidelines (the “outside-in”). In a context of inconsistent, ad hoc “rules”, unclear or contradictory communication, punishment for “infractions”, and the elimination of relational agency, patients like Brianna and Jake are forced to navigate an uncertain landscape, enacting their intimate and sexual relationalities in subversive, secretive, and potentially perilous ways. Brianna and Jake, like many of the forensic mental healthcare patients we spoke to, articulated a relationship between their intimate relationality and their recovery. For Brianna, the enforced hiatus in sexual activity with anyone but Trevian had made her feel “clean”, and her dancing gave her purpose and made her feel good; for Jake, sex and emotional intimacy supported his emerging sense of self, which underpins positive mental health and contributes to recovery (Shepherd et al., 2016). That patient perspectives on this link between sexuality and recovery are largely missing from accounts of both relational security and recovery does not mean that intimate and sexual relationality has no role in either of these; rather, its role is obscured by a culture of sexual prohibition and pervasive discourses of risk and appropriateness (Ravenhill et al., 2020). Insights from people like Brianna and Jake reveal that at least some patients feel sexual, enact intimate and sexual relationality, and experience (and can articulate) the connection between their sexuality and their mental health, yet official guidance on relational security, including its therapeutic potential, almost entirely overlooks the intimate and sexual relationships many patients engage in with themselves and others. Providing “purposeful” therapy, understanding patient dynamics, and knowing patients’ inner and outer worlds are fundamental for maintaining relational security (Allen, 2015); however, without an understanding of patients’ feelings and practices around sexuality, romance, and emotional and physical intimacy, it is hard to see how this can be achieved. The key to maintaining relational security, in terms of both risk-reduction and clinical recovery, must be the broadening of interpretations of the concept, to incorporate patients’ intimate relational desires and needs. The provision and implementation of clear policies should be underpinned by a more nuanced understanding of relational security, based on the principles that ward safety is a shared endeavour between facility management, clinical staff, ward staff, and patients alike and that sexuality must form part of initial assessments and be addressed directly in care planning. Policies that involve patients in the conversation, where the potential for sexuality to contribute to recovery is explored *alongside* considerations of risk, would demystify patient sexuality, bring it to the open, and offer a framework for staff to work safely and positively with their patients on all issues relating to intimate and sexual relationality.

Acknowledgements Thank you to the people who shared their experiences as part of this research. This research was funded by a Wellcome Seed Award in Humanities and Social Science (award number 207925/Z/17/Z).

References

Alden, L. (1978). Factor analysis of the Ward Atmosphere Scale. *Journal of Consulting and Clinical Psychology, 46*, 175–176. https://doi.org/10.1037/0022-006X.46.1.175

Allen, E. (2015). *See think act: Relational security in secure mental health services*. Royal College of Psychiatrists. Retrieved from https://tinyurl.com/mr452ehk

Bartlett, P., Mantovani, N., Cratsley, K., Dillon, C., & Eastman, N. (2010). "You may kiss the bride, but you may not open your mouth when you do so": Policies concerning sex, marriage, and relationships in English forensic psychiatric facilities. *Liverpool Law Review, 31*, 155–176. https://doi.org/10.1007/s10991-010-9078-5

Boden, Z., & Eatough, V. (2014). Understanding more fully: A multimodal hermeneutic-phenomenological approach. *Qualitative Research in Psychology, 11*, 160–177. https://doi.org/10.1080/14780887.2013.853854

Brown, S. D., Reavey, P., Kanyeredzi, A., & Batty, R. (2014). Transformations of self and sexuality: Psychologically modified experiences in the context of forensic mental health. *Health, 18*, 240–260. https://doi.org/10.1177/1363459313497606

Care Quality Commission. (2018). *Sexual safety on mental health wards*. Care Quality Commission.

Caudill, W. (1958). The psychiatric hospital as a small society. *Harvard University Press*. https://doi.org/10.4159/harvard.9780674598737

Chester, V., & Morgan, W. (2012). Relational security in secure services: Summary of findings from a literature review. *Quality Network for Forensic Mental Health Services Newsletter, 20*, 10–14.

Chester, V., Alexander, R. T., & Morgan, W. (2017). Measuring relational security in forensic mental health services. *BJPsych Bulletin, 41*, 358–363. https://doi.org/10.1192/pb.bp.116.055509

Clarke, C., Lumbard, D., Sambrook, S., & Kerr, K. (2016). What does recovery mean to a forensic mental health patient? A systematic review and narrative synthesis of the qualitative literature. *The Journal of Forensic Psychiatry & Psychology, 27*, 38–54. https://doi.org/10.1080/14789949.2015.1102311

Curtis, S., Gesler, W., Wood, V., Spencer, I., Mason, J., Close, H., & Reilly, J. (2013). Compassionate containment? Balancing technical safety and therapy in the design of psychiatric wards. *Social Science & Medicine, 97*, 201–209. https://doi.org/10.1016/j.socscimed.2013.06.015

Dein, K. E., & Williams, P. S. (2008). Relationships between residents in secure psychiatric units: Are safety and sensitivity really incompatible? *The Psychiatrist, 32*, 284–287. https://doi.org/10.1192/pb.bp.106.011478

Dein, K. E., Williams, P. S., & Dein, S. (2007). The ethnic bias in the application of the Mental Health Act of 1983. *Advances in Psychiatric Treatment, 13*, 350–357. https://doi.org/10.1192/apt.bp.107.003582

Dein, K. E., Williams, P. S., Volkonskaia, I., Kanyeredzi, A., Reavey, P., & Leavey, G. (2016). Examining professionals' perspectives on sexuality for service users of a forensic psychiatry unit. *International Journal of Law and Psychiatry, 44*, 15–23. https://doi.org/10.1016/j.ijlp.2015.08.027

Doyle, P., Quayle, E., & Newman, E. (2017). Social climate in forensic mental health settings: A systematic review of qualitative studies. *Aggression and Violent Behavior, 36*, 118–136. https://doi.org/10.1016/j/avb.2017.06.008

Drennan, G., & Alden, D. (2012). Preface. In G. Drennan & D. Alden (Eds.), *Secure recovery: Approaches to recovery in forensic mental health settings* (pp. viii–xv). Routledge.

Fuchs, T. (2013). The phenomenology of affectivity. In K. W. M. Fulford, M. Davies, R. G. T. Gipps, G. Graham, J. Z. Sadler, G. Stanghellini, & T. Thornton (Eds.), *The Oxford handbook of philosophy and psychiatry* (pp. 612–631). Oxford University Press. https://doi.org/10.1093/oxfordhb/9780199579563.013.0038

Hare Duke, L., Furtado, V., Guo, B., & Völlm, B. A. (2018). Long-stay in forensic-psychiatric care in the UK. *Social Psychiatry and Psychiatric Epidemiology, 53*, 313–321. https://doi.org/10.1007/s00127-017-1473-y

Hunter, K. M., & Ahmed, A. O. (2016). Sexuality and sexual health. In N. N. Singh, J. W. Barber, & S. Van Sant (Eds.), *Handbook of recovery in inpatient psychiatry* (pp. 59–79). Springer.

Jacob, J. D., & Holmes, D. (2011). The culture of fear: Expanding the concept of risk in forensic psychiatric nursing. *International Journal of Culture and Mental Health, 4*, 106–115. https://doi.org/10.1080/17542863.2010.519123

Kennedy, H. G. (2002). Therapeutic uses of security: mapping forensic mental health services by stratifying risk. *Advances in Psychiatric Treatment, 8*, 433–443.

Laithwaite, H., & Gumley, A. (2007). Sense of self, adaptation and recovery in patients with psychosis in a forensic NHS setting. *Clinical Psychology & Psychotherapy: An International Journal of Theory & Practice, 14*, 302–316. https://doi.org/10.1002/cpp.538

McCann, E. (2000). The expression of sexuality in people with psychosis: Breaking the taboos. *Journal of Advanced Nursing, 32*, 132–138. https://doi.org/10.1046/j.1365-2648.2000.01452.x

Moos, R. H. (1967). The differential effect of ward settings on psychiatric patients. *Journal of Nervous and Mental Disease, 14S*, 272–283.

Moos, R. H., & Houts, P. S. (1968). Assessment of the social atmospheres of psychiatric wards. *Journal of Abnormal Psychology, 73*, 595–604.

NHS. (2022). *Data dictionary*. https://www.datadictionary.nhs.uk/

NHS England. (2016). *The five year forward view for mental health*. Retrieved from https://www.england.nhs.uk/wp-content/uploads/2016/02/Mental-Health-Taskforce-FYFV-final.pdf

Quinn, C., & Happell, B. (2016). Supporting the sexual intimacy needs of patients in a longer stay inpatient forensic setting. *Perspectives in Psychiatric Care, 52*, 239–247. https://doi.org/10.1111/ppc.12123

Ravenhill, J. P., Poole, J., Brown, S. D., & Reavey, P. (2020). Sexuality, risk, and organisational misbehavior in a secure mental healthcare facility in England. *Culture, Health & Sexuality, 22*, 1382–1397. https://doi.org/10.1080/13691058.2019.1683900

Reavey, P., & Brown, S. D. (2021). Visual Data. In E. Lyons & A. Coyle (Eds.), *Analysing qualitative data in psychology* (pp. 100–121). Sage.

Reavey, P, Poole, J., Corrigall, R., Zundel, T., Byford, S., Sarhane, M., Taylor, E., Ivens, J., & Ougrin, D. (2017). The ward as an emotional ecology: Adolescent experiences of managing mental health and distress in psychiatric inpatient settings. *Health and Place, 46*, 210–218. https://doi.org/10.1016/j.healthplace.2017.05.008

Reavey, P., Brown, S. D., Ravenhill, J. P., Boden-Stuart, Z., & Ciarlo, D. (2022). Choreographies of sexual safety and liminality: Forensic mental health and the limits of recovery. SSM Mental Health, 2, 100090. https://doi.org/10.1016/j.ssmmh.2022.100090

Royal College of Psychiatrists. (2017). *Sexual boundaries in clinical practice.* Royal College of Psychiatrists. Retrieved from https://bit.ly/2p0Hmyg

Royal College of Psychiatrists. (2022). *Relational security explorer.* Retrieved from https://tinyurl.com/yckp8sdf

Ruane, J., & Hayter, M. (2008). Nurses' attitudes towards sexual relationships between patients in high security psychiatric hospitals in England: An exploratory qualitative study. *International Journal of Nursing Studies, 45*, 1731–1741. https://doi.org/10.1016/j.ijnurstu.2008.06.003

Schalast, N., Redies, M., Collins, M., Stacey, J., & Howells, K. (2008). EssenCES, a short questionnaire for assessing the social climate of forensic psychiatric wards. *Criminal Behaviour and Mental Health, 18*, 49–58. https://doi.org/10.1002/cbm.677

Series, L. (2014). Sex, capacity and forensic cotton wool: IM v LM [2014] EWCA Civ 37. *Journal of Social Welfare & Family Law, 36*, 317–319. https://doi.org/10.1080/09649069.2014.933594

Shepherd, G., Boardman, J., & Slade, M. (2008). *Making recovery a reality.* Sainsbury Centre for Mental Health.

Shepherd, A., Doyle, M., Sanders, C., & Shaw, J. (2016). Personal recovery within forensic settings–Systematic review and meta-synthesis of qualitative methods studies. *Criminal Behaviour and Mental Health, 26*, 59–75. https://doi.org/10.1002/cbm.1966

Stern, D. N. (2010). *Forms of vitality: Exploring dynamic experience in psychology, the arts, psychotherapy and development.* Oxford University Press.

Tighe, J., & Gudjonsson, G. H. (2012). See, Think, Act Scale: Preliminary development and validation of a measure of relational security in medium- and low-secure units. *The Journal of Forensic Psychiatry & Psychology, 23*, 184–199. https://doi.org/10.1080/14789949.2012.671336

Tonkin, M. (2016). A review of questionnaire measures for assessing the social climate in prisons and forensic psychiatric hospitals. *International Journal of Offender Therapy and Comparative Criminology, 60*, 1376–1405. https://doi.org/10.1177/0306624X15578834

Part V

New Directions: Building a Relational Approach to Distress and Recovery

14

The Development of a Relational Practice Movement

Rex Haigh and Nick Benefield

Currently, narrow industrialised models of public service interventions ignore many factors in the wider system, including the need to take a broader approach to the complexity of working with others. The powerful effect of managerialism and market competitiveness combine to produce a milieu in which human values and relationships are not explicitly prioritised: the experience of public services is increasingly impoverished and alienating for those providing or receiving them. In the current situation, professionals face the risk of losing their capacity to maintain a relational basis to the work.

This chapter outlines the process that led to the recognition of this 'relational practice' deficit, its definition and recognition, the change needed, the intention of our campaign and the underlying theoretical framework. We call for change in the training and practice of all professional and ancillary staff working in public services. Commissioning will need to drive these changes if future public services are to be fit for twenty-first-century requirements. To implement this, we have been

R. Haigh • N. Benefield (✉)
Independent, London, UK
e-mail: nick.benefield@icloud.com

Z. Boden-Stuart, M. Larkin (eds.), *Relationships and Mental Health*,
https://doi.org/10.1007/978-3-031-50047-3_14

coordinating a small professional campaign over the last few years and intend to launch an accompanying manifesto in mid-2023.

Introduction

The English Department of Health's National Personality Disorder Programme (2003–2011) was launched with the publication of *No Longer a Diagnosis of Exclusion* (NIMHE, 2003) and closed with the publication of a practice handbook (Winifred Bolton et al., 2014) and a qualitative service evaluation (Wilson & Haigh, 2011). The whole process became a vehicle for the identification, research and development of 'relational practice' (Haigh & Benefield, 2020).

This was achieved through establishing a range of different pilot projects across the country (Haigh, 2007), studying them with a mixed methods research programme (Crawford et al., 2007) and implementing a 'training escalator' to develop a workforce with suitable knowledge, understanding and attitudes (NIMHE, 2003). The programme also supported the development of a rigorous but relational and values-based process for identifying, measuring and ultimately accrediting best practice, through the Royal College of Psychiatrists Centre for Quality Improvements 'Enabling Environments' programme (Haigh et al., 2012).

This was all to provide innovative solutions to what was seen as the 'burden' of 'personality disorders' (PD) in community and inpatient mental health services (Soeteman et al., 2008). This was traditionally seen as a 'hard-to-reach' population who were often excluded from mainstream services. People with this diagnosis were often disliked as 'patients'; working with them was seen as difficult and inappropriate by many staff, because they did not have 'proper mental illnesses' (Lewis & Appleby, 1988).

Rationale

When human development is disrupted, the psychological, social and economic consequences can reach into every area of an individual's personal and social world, resulting in alienated and chaotic lives and repercussions throughout their communities. The causes and consequences are largely relational. They may include child abuse, inadequate parenting, failed attachment, trauma or emotional deprivation. The causes can also be social: material poverty, or the poverty of expectation that leaves individuals feeling powerless to have any impact on the world in which they live.

Over-riding differences in class and educational advantage confer some with strong constitutions—or a range of poorly understood 'protective factors'—which may be sufficient to enable them to withstand the impact of these environmental failures and emerge from their early experience to live what appear to be thriving and healthy lives (Bellis et al., 2016). However, very many end up in a situation where they are excluded from mainstream society, rejected by those who might be able to help them and destined to live without the happiness and fulfilment that most of us would consider just—and expect for ourselves and our families.

These individuals, and often their families, have little psychological sense of their place amongst others or where they fit into society. School, working lives and almost any pro-social relationships are difficult or impossible to establish and sustain. They experience the world as a hostile, unhelpful, threatening or undermining environment, living in a marginalised underclass with high levels of substance misuse, self-harm, criminality and suffering severe, enduring and disabling mental distress (Horn et al., 2007). People in this situation will often use a considerable range of statutory services to little benefit (Coid et al., 2009).

If our systems could respond in a relational way, our experience in working with 'personality disorder' services and systems shows that many obstacles, obstructions and conflicts could be prevented. This applies at the individual level (when those seeking service input feel respected and not overpowered by the professional they consult); service level (where those working in the service have meaningful engagement with their task, believe in what they are doing and can operate from a position of authenticity and wanting to help—rather than by just following a rulebook); organisational level (these principles need to be prioritised and not overruled by role hierarchies or inflexible procedures); and political level (so that policymakers in different areas can develop a shared understanding of how changes in this direction will lead to greater efficiency and satisfaction, for both service users and providers).

Contextual History

The phenomenon of 'personality disorder' first caught public and government attention following the 1996 murders of Lin and Megan Russell and the attempted murder of Josie Russell, by Michael Stone in Kent (Kent County Council, 2006). This led to what became known as the Dangerous People with Severe Personality Disorder (DSPD) programme (Maden, 2006). The political objective was to research into improved management of high-risk offenders whose risk to others was linked to their diagnosis of personality disorder. The outcome was the piloting of new assessment and treatment services based in prisons, NHS secure services and community forensic teams. This programme provided a joint financial investment by the Department of Health and Home Office. As part of the policy plan it made a commitment to improve mainstream community mental health and social care services for those failed by existing services because of their identified 'personality disorder' presentation. This then became established as the National Personality Disorder Programme in 2003.

At about the same time, a self-help organisation called Borderline UK was set up with a Millennium Lottery grant; it was headed and run by people with lived experience of personality disorder, with some support from sympathetic professionals. There was, and still is, considerable controversy about the use of the 'personality disorder' label itself. In terms of provision, many anguished voices claimed unhelpful and harmful treatment from statutory services (Castillo, 2003; Robinson & Cox, 2006; Sibbald, 2020).

Recognising these unmet needs, the Department of Health set up two working groups to prepare a policy implementation document on strategic changes that might help. In 2003 *Personality Disorder, No Longer a Diagnosis of Exclusion* (NIMHE, 2003), with clear evidence on what service users were asking for, was published alongside the *Breaking the Cycle of Rejection: Personality Disorder Capabilities Framework* (NIMHE, 2003), which was a guide on workforce development and establishing a training escalator relevant to all disciplines and levels of seniority. A National Personality Disorder Development Programme, for services in the community, was established. The three stated aims of the national programme were (1) to produce innovative service developments, (2) to have a national evaluation of the new services and (3) to implement national regional training developments.

Several new services were established in 2004, and two years later, a national learning network was established as a forum, which was attended by service users, staff and managers from all 11 of the new community pilot projects. The discussions were fertile ground for sharing best practice, and new knowledge, as well as the inevitable obstructions and difficulties. The programme was also evaluated (Crawford et al., 2007). An important part of the programme was the extensive involvement and partnership with service users, now also known as 'experts by experience' ('XBXs' or 'EBEs') or 'people with lived experience'.

The most influential product of the partnership, and of the cooperative and trusting relationship between professionals and those with lived experience, was the Knowledge and Understanding Framework ('KUF') training. It started in 2008, with Emergence plus three partners: the Open University, Tavistock and Portman NHS Trust, and Nottingham's Mental Health Institute. There were three levels of training on the 'career escalator': the awareness level training—which had been delivered to nearly 200,000 people by the end of the mid-2010s; a stand-alone BSc course which later became Continuing Professional Development (CPD) modules; and an MSc delivered across four centres. The principle of the KUF training is that it is co-produced at all levels—from writing the material to recording videos, the online content and the delivery. For example, the three face-to-face days on the awareness training are always delivered by a lived experience practitioner partnered with a sympathetic clinician, who had been through a train-the-trainers programme together.

Three important government documents were published in 2009: the *Recognising Complexity* commissioning guidance for personality disorder services (Department of Health, 2009) and the National Institute for Mental Health in England (NICE) guidelines on Borderline Personality Disorder (NICE, CG78, 2009b) and Antisocial Personality Disorder (NICE, 2009a). These strengthened the understanding of how different presentations would need specifically designed services and provided commissioners with a model for developing them for people with what is now sometimes called 'complex emotional needs' or 'complex trauma'. At its peak, the new community PD services were only covering 12% of the English population: questions were being asked about what existed for the other 88%. By 2011, the effects of the economic crisis led to the community programme being closed.

However, following the recommendations of the 2009 Bradley Report (Bradley, 2009), much of the learning from the community programme was incorporated into the joint Ministry of Justice/NHS Offender Personality Disorder Programme in 2011. This programme has seen the biggest development of sustainable services within the criminal justice pathways for high-risk offenders. These assessment and treatment services include prison-based therapeutic communities (Shuker & Newton, 2008), specialist Psychologically Informed Planned Environments (PIPEs) (Benefield et al., 2017) and numerous prison units joining the programme to become 'Enabling Environments' (Haigh et al., 2012). For these men and women, who have complex needs and have histories of relational difficulties, we have provided innovative interventions and improved relational environments. In doing so we have developed our understanding of relational practice and the need to focus on the provision of reliable, consistent longer-term relational experience.

The community programme finished with two publications and a number of other indirect developments. The first is a qualitative evaluation of all 11 community pilot projects, *Innovation in Action* (Wilson & Haigh, 2011) which recognised the importance of the *quality of relationships* and described many common factors and whole-system features ('general therapeutic factors') of what was to become 'relational practice'.

The second publication was *Meeting the Challenge, Making a Difference*, a handbook for working in various settings where mental health is a factor (from homelessness hostels and social care settings to psychiatric hospitals, for example). It is a user-friendly, accessible and practical guide, based on all that had been learnt from the pilot projects (Winifred Bolton et al., 2014). Linked work at the Royal College of Psychiatrists Centre for Quality Improvement, from 2007 onwards, these publications led to an accreditation process for 'Enabling Environments', which was based on ten relationship-based values. The ten standards represented the core features of any relational practice environment together with a process through which they could be established, recognised and sustained (Royal College of Psychiatrists, 2016).

A 'Relational Practice Movement'

Widespread understanding and implementation of relational practice is required for the future delivery of public services. This will involve due attention to the quality of relationships necessary for effective and meaningful human exchange. It is likely that the health of all involved, support for their resilience and effectiveness of the work are contingent upon the quality of the relational environment in which they work. In any pathway of engagement between an individual and the services they use, the foundation of that engagement is a relational one. This requires that the exchange is respectful and personalised and takes account of the previous experience and present position of all participants. The intention is to build a productive relationship between those who use services and those who provide them, in the context of shared ownership and effective personal agency, with an understanding of any intrinsic power differences.

This is important because the provision of education, good mental and physical health, social and criminal justice care and support is not provided purely by the system of delivery, but also provided by the quality and collective understanding of those professionals engaged with this delivery. A healthy workforce must not be stressed to the point of burnout, lost to sick leave or to leaving their various professions. Rather, a healthy workforce is one in which people enjoy their relational contacts with clients and colleagues and feel valued and directly involved in a shared endeavour that is inherently meaningful, worthwhile and interesting. However, relationships cannot be prescribed, or pre-determined, to be positive. Relational practice is not a definitive solution, and working in this way must acknowledge how future relationships are often determined by the quality and problems of participants' previous relationships. Managing, or just enduring, difficult relationships is an unavoidable part of the work.

We now have 18 years of clinical practice, lived experience and evidence from the developing field of personality disorder, meaning it is now possible to identify and deliver the service design and workforce development needed for relational practice. As yet there is only an established policy in specialist areas of criminal justice and their mental health services. What is required is a movement whose campaigning objective is to make the case for designing, staffing and developing relational practice, at all levels, in a range of public service settings.

Expectations of reasonable human rights in a public service system are all based on a relational understanding that there should be:

- Access to meet need
- Respect and dignity
- Understanding and empathy
- Empowerment and participation
- Consistency and informed choice

This requires all staff to be trained, skilled and supported to understand and provide a meaningful relational response.

Definition of Relational Practice

In many situations within public services, those using them are vulnerable, have little or no personal authority or support to help make their case, and feel frightened. If they have needed various different services, or had numerous unsuccessful interactions, they may have little trust in the services' ability to help them. The same can also be true for people without such marked vulnerabilities, who do have personal resources with adequate strength and determination, but find themselves lost in complex systems, major parts of which are only accessible online, and for whom it seems impossible to have a rational conversation with a human being who can help.

These negative expectations can be ameliorated or exacerbated by the quality of relationship between the person seeking a service and the person (and organisation) providing it. A mechanical and purely transactional interaction where the provider only reads a script or asks standard questions in a disinterested way is likely to add to any bad feelings of isolation, helplessness and possibly anger. Alternatively, a human and friendly response which shows some friendliness, warmth and perhaps compassion is much likelier to lead to a useful conversation with an outcome of hope (or at least being understood) for the recipient and satisfaction of a job well done for the provider.

Many policies, at all levels, translate into restrictions and obstacles that set a tone of low expectations and likely disappointment and conflict. For example, 'zero tolerance' notices of violence in a hospital ward should never be necessary; 'zero tolerance' mathematically equates to 'infinite intolerance', which feels to be the direction in which many things are heading. By rigidly enforcing 'thin rules' (Daston, 2022), discretion is disallowed and both provider and recipient of services are disempowered.

Our observations of the substantial difference that 'relational practice' can make in some of the most challenging settings and situations—such as with people diagnosed with severe personality disorder in prison settings—have led us to see that this way of working is often seriously lacking in many other public service settings.

What follows is a first definition to pin down some essential qualities of what we have observed. It will require revision as definitive evidence emerges from more rigorous research:

> *Relational Practice gives priority to interpersonal relationships, in both external and internal aspects. It is the foundation upon which effective interventions are made, and it forms the conditions for a healthy relational environment. It requires relationships based on reliability, consistency, curiosity, flexibility, and*

authenticity; an enabling and facilitating attitude; and an understanding of the conscious and unconscious lives of individuals and groups in their social field. (Benefield N & Haigh R, public lecture, Univeristy of Central Lancashire, 27 January 2020)

Research and Evidence Supporting Relational Practice

Although the research does not use the term 'relational practice', there is a growing evidence base that these approaches have positive benefits and outcomes in prison populations (e.g. see Auty & Liebling, 2020). A relevant National Institute of Health Research (NIHR)-funded study of service user perspectives on current provision clearly identified the central importance of relational practice and labelled it thus (Trevillion et al., 2021). Further studies are underway and soon to be published (anticipated in 2023), including a literature search and systematic review; a Delphi exercise is then planned. More comprehensive studies on implementation are also under consideration.

Recognition of Relational Practice

Figure 14.1 shows some of the current activities in four areas of the relational practice movement: policy, training, research and campaigning. The initiatives with the most anticipated impact are those outlined in bold.

The 'Enabling Environments' programme was started at the Royal College of Psychiatrists Centre for Quality Improvement in 2007 (Haigh et al., 2012). The impetus was to produce a set of values derived from work undertaken in the previous five years with the 'Community of Communities' quality network and from workshops with professionals and organisations in fields which saw 'working with relationships' as a central principle of their practice.

Ten 'values', each a single word (Fig. 14.2), were thus defined to describe what were felt to be the most salient features of working in a

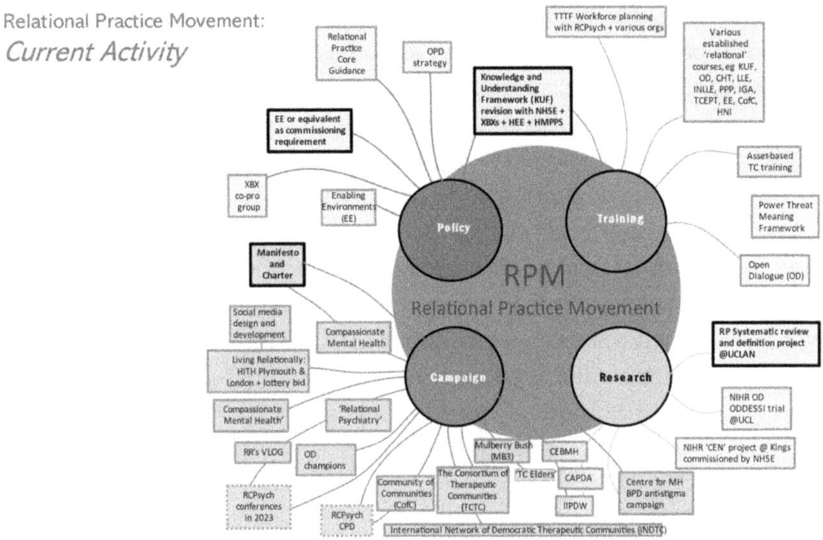

Fig. 14.1 Organisations and activities identified as involved in relational practice (mid-2022)

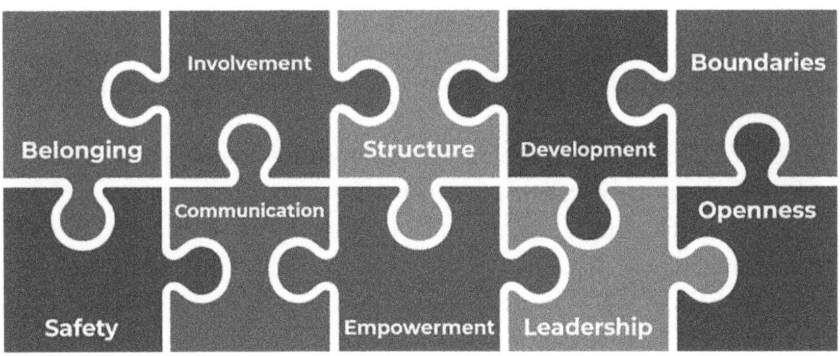

Fig. 14.2 The ten values by which the Enabling Environments project recognises relational practice

'relational' way. A short phrase was then assigned to each of the ten values, as concisely as possible, to describe an expectation or standard linked to that value. These ten standards are measurable against criteria which demonstrate that they are being met; each standard has three or four examples of such criteria which are published with the standards. However, participating services are also able to use other criteria, if they can justify how they demonstrate that the standard is being met. The whole process is planned and operated in a process which emphasises engagement and collaboration rather than compliance and inspection.

The process of recognition and accreditation is formalised through the submission of a portfolio of evidence, standardised questionnaires and a visit by a team of experts. Production of the portfolio is a substantial piece of work and requires engagement and collaboration—in other words, relational practice—to undertake it. The results are reviewed by a Royal College Accreditation Panel and may result in full accreditation for three years—or recommendations for changes needed to achieve it.

The ten values and standards are:

BELONGING: The nature and quality of relationships are of primary importance.
BOUNDARIES: There are expectations of behaviour and processes to maintain and review them.
COMMUNICATION: It is recognised that people communicate in different ways.
DEVELOPMENT: There are opportunities to be spontaneous and try new things.
INVOLVEMENT: Everyone shares responsibility for the environment.
SAFETY: Support is available for everyone.
STRUCTURE: Engagement and purposeful activity are actively encouraged.
EMPOWERMENT: Power and authority are open to discussion.
LEADERSHIP: Leadership takes responsibility for the environment being enabling.
OPENNESS: External relationships are sought and valued.

Details of how services using relational practice principles can be recognised and accredited, and more details, are available from the Royal College of Psychiatrists (Royal College of Psychiatrists, 2016).

This framework has been most extensively used in criminal justice settings, with services from various other sectors also achieving accreditation—as a quality mark to demonstrate, amongst other valuable characteristics, that they have relational work at the heart of their operations.

Theoretical Framework Underpinning Relational Practice

The relational practice movement is based on a model of human and emotional development (Haigh & Benefield, 2019) which draws on a wide range of basic concepts with relevance to 'relationship' and explicit theories of need and causation of behaviours and emotions. This embraces the fields of psychoanalysis, group analysis, social sciences, education, life-course development, neurosciences, management and organisational dynamics.

At its core, emotional development is an overlapping but chronological sequence of required human experiences based on psychoanalytic concepts of *attachment* (Bowlby, 2008) and *containment* (Bion, 1985; Winnicott, 1965), group analytic theory of *communication* and *inclusion* (Foulkes, 1983), and social psychology writings on responsible *agency* (Pearce & Pickard, 2013). The quality of the environment in which these happen can be described as one of belonging, safety, openness, inclusion and empowerment (Haigh, 2013).

The wider human development model (Fig. 14.3) extends this with a simple underlying premise: that a vast range of internal and external factors determine the lives we will all lead. The fact that it is a 'vast range' makes it difficult to summarise and group them into a simple diagram or description. Also, the whole range of factors is almost impossible to precisely define, and the fixed and continuous interactions between them all create an almost infinite number of paths for personality development, as well as life outcome and what we all leave behind. The 'outcome', perhaps defined as 'what our life is like', can perhaps be best seen as an emergent property of a complex and possibly chaotic system.

The synthesis behind the model was developed over several years by an iterative consultation process with experts-by-experience, clinicians and

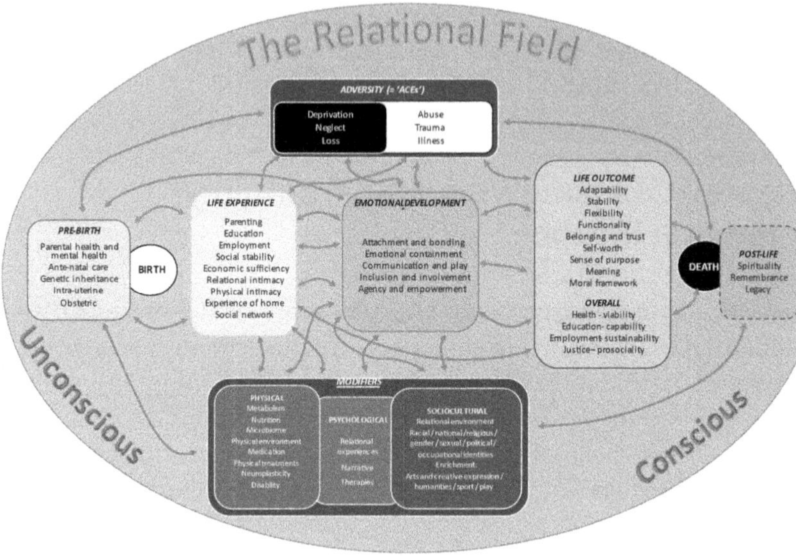

Fig. 14.3 The complex interplay of numerous variables in human development

academics at a UK-based annual conference. It starts before birth and finishes after death; the major areas between the two are emotional development, life experience and life outcome. All these areas can be influenced by adversity—by omission or commission—and modified by a range of 'bio-psycho-social' factors. Many of these adversities are covered by the increasing use of the concept of 'trauma-informed practice'. All these elements and interactions are seen to exist in a relational field, part of which is experienced consciously (and therefore subject to a degree of rational understanding) but much is unconscious (or autonomic) and therefore not explicable by the straightforward logic of cause and effect.

Levels of Relational Practice

As clearly identified ideas, principles and values emerged, the concept of relational practice gained greater definition, and a framework for how it could be implemented across a wider field of public and human services emerged. It can be argued that the root of many prominent breakdowns in delivery of public services can be seen as a failure of relational practice—at individual, practice or organisation levels.

Relational practice is predicated on the recognition of the fundamental importance of the relational field and that all professional work requires good quality relationships. Clearly, this goes beyond an understanding using only biomedical psychiatry (Thomas et al., 2005); the model proposed here also goes beyond the widely taught and used one of a biopsychosocial approach (Engel, 1980), which proposed that all three aspects (biological, psychological and social) need to be considered in consideration of health and illness. Figure 14.3 also shows that the interplay also needs to include political, economic, ecological and deeply felt spiritual and cultural factors. All need to be considered part of an individual's relational field, from early socialisation to the physical and mental consequences of advancing debility and impending death.

The facilitation of development leading to a healthy pro-social life is a pre-requisite of practice based on establishing, maintaining and using relationships in all areas of life: personal and professional. Although 'relational practice' most clearly relates to professional life, it has an underpinning that is likely to be inauthentic if it were only to exist in one's work. This could even be seen as the antithesis of 'professional armour' with which some professionals protect themselves from the necessity of engaging at a level of intimacy that they wish to avoid. In medicine, this is akin to a doctor 'hiding behind the white coat' as opposed to 'having a good bedside manner'.

A comprehensive understanding of relationality does require the use of the psychoanalytic concepts of unconscious and irrational processes—as they affect feelings, attitudes and behaviours—and the many other human factors represented in the model. However, the day-to-day work of relational practice is actually very ordinary, and for many people, probably much easier to do than to maintain a pseudo-professional attitude bound by implicit, or sometimes explicit, rules of conduct, speech, dress, ritual, hierarchy and other power dynamics. It is about the authenticity of being able to 'be oneself' in professional relationships, which will sometimes need to include difficult decisions, painful actions and anxious uncertainty. Working in this way requires informed senior leadership that recognises relational principles and practice, which includes being compassionate, tolerant, flexible and available. Acknowledgement of a society's changing norms is also required—being relational in the 1960s was probably very different from the 1990s, or today. What is permissible in different eras, and to different generations of individuals, cannot be ignored; to do so is likely to lead to acrimonious misunderstanding, and the very antithesis of the openness and safety required. Also, the form and acceptability of relational practice are not going to be the same in different parts of the world.

The ability to work in this way will clearly vary between individuals: to some it will come naturally (and is how they have always worked); to others it may be a new and unexpectedly enjoyable way of operating; to some it will be feared, avoided and resisted. Training, support and encouragement are likely to be needed for many. For the work that requires a high level of relational practice, perhaps such as certain forms of psychotherapy, dealing with customer complaints or the teaching of children, it is probably best to select out those who are likely to find it too difficult before they begin. In many positions requiring some degree of relationality, standard working practice—such as good induction, team-building and emphasis on collaboration and cooperation rather than authoritarian hierarchy and rivalry—may well be enough. In such environments, it is likely to already exist in a sustainable way.

Structurally, relational practice needs to exist at several levels: the individual one-to-one encounter; the group or team within which practitioners are working; and the wider organisation which is responsible for delivering that work—and the relationship between it and other organisations, as well as the political or commissioning structures within which the organisation exists.

Personal Qualities

Each individual's capacity to participate in good quality relationships requires consideration of their personal and emotional capabilities in delivering professional tasks. Failure to do so can undermine the effectiveness of their professional role and risk burnout or harmful mental health consequences and can have a negative impact on others, including service users. Although all interpersonal work requires relational understanding, recruitment to roles requiring specific relational skills needs to consider criteria to identify relevant vulnerabilities and capacities in more depth.

One-to-One Relationships

The *quality of relationship* is a measure of the way in which relationships are established, maintained, developed and concluded. *Establishing* a one-to-one relationship requires an attitude of genuineness and authenticity, based on a consideration of how it must feel to be in the other's place. It is often helped by behaviour demonstrating openness and informality; understanding any power differential and the intended purpose is essential. Speaking with a prescribed form of words and working purely from a decision tree are not sufficient in themselves. *Developing* the relationship is important in relationships which will endure over time. This requires different actions depending on the intervals between contacts and the duration of engagement. The intention is to produce a feeling of safety within which confidence can be established. A sense of playfulness may help. *Maintaining* the relationship needs both reliability and flexibility. The experience of being fully heard requires a particular quality of listening and willingness to hear. It must include an understanding of the conscious and unconscious impact of the emotional content and our way of processing it. The purpose of the relationship is kept in mind, and boundaries are understood. Cancelled appointments and change of personnel, particularly at short notice, are harmful to relational continuity and organisational trustworthiness. Disagreements, breakdowns and ruptures in the relationship need to be mended wherever possible. Ending all relationships has a significance which needs consideration, particularly those of longer duration or importance. Endings are best when agreed and accepted and should be based on principles of reliability and consistency. Endings are transitions which may have problematic associations for those who have had earlier difficulties with attachment and separations. Missing or avoiding an ending should not happen.

Group Culture

One-to-one relationships always exist in the context of a wider group. The group environment needs to facilitate the conditions for healthy one-to-one relating while recognising the constraints of different settings. Belonging and connection form the basis of engagement and identity; involvement and inclusion are needed to feel part of something and to take a participating role; boundaries and limits are required to provide an experience of psychological containment, within which thinking together is more possible; safety and confidence arise from a psychosocially designed environment; authenticity and communication provide a way to give behaviour meaning; openness and transparency reduce suspiciousness, support honesty and allow the development of trust. Spontaneity and flexibility can provide an opportunity for the exploration of imaginative and innovative ideas and thinking; ownership, responsibility and power create conditions for mutual control, shared accountability and self-determination; personal agency and freedom allow individuals to maintain their own mind and have freedom to make choices. All relational environments require clarity of purpose and leadership to ensure that a relational environment is maintained.

Organisational Culture

Service pathways involve a range of organisational settings. Each organisation will have its own culture relating to its primary purpose, but it will need to establish an environment in which relational practice can be sustained. For services and teams, the setting requires physical facilities and organisational conditions to optimise interpersonal relational life; the leadership needs to understand and be committed to establishing and maintaining a relational environment as central to healthy working conditions and staff well-being, as well as improved effectiveness and satisfaction, with fewer complaints. Arrangements for support and supervision must be integral to the organisation's design. An atmosphere of curiosity ensures a reflective approach to all aspects of the service environment and enrichment of the organisational culture reaches beyond the primary task by providing experience and allowing access to imaginative and creative experiences.

For workforce development, all organisations and teams in public sector pathways need to have a relational practice training strategy. This will cover awareness, understanding, skills, and the recruitment and selection of staff, which needs to continue as part of professional growth. Service-specific elements of relational practice training will be required in different contexts. Depending on the organisational context, this may include the risk to self and others, attitude to rules and issues of discretion.

Conclusion

Relational practice is a way of working that was identified and highlighted through the implementation of the Department of Health's 'National Personality Disorder Programme (2003–11). Its relevance is much wider than 'personality disorder', or mental health, or indeed all health services. Human development is something we all experience (Haigh & Benefield, 2019), and healthy development forms the basis of requirements needed to produce suitable therapeutic cultures and working practices (Haigh, 2000, 2004; Royal College of Psychiatrists, 2016). An understanding of the relational field provides a working understanding of human exchange that should guide the daily practice of public sector tasks.

This work must continue, develop and extend as research and evidence emerges to demonstrate improved professionals' working culture and increased effectiveness—with improved user outcomes. This is relevant across all sectors of public service, and the manifesto's strategic plan is shown in Fig. 14.4.

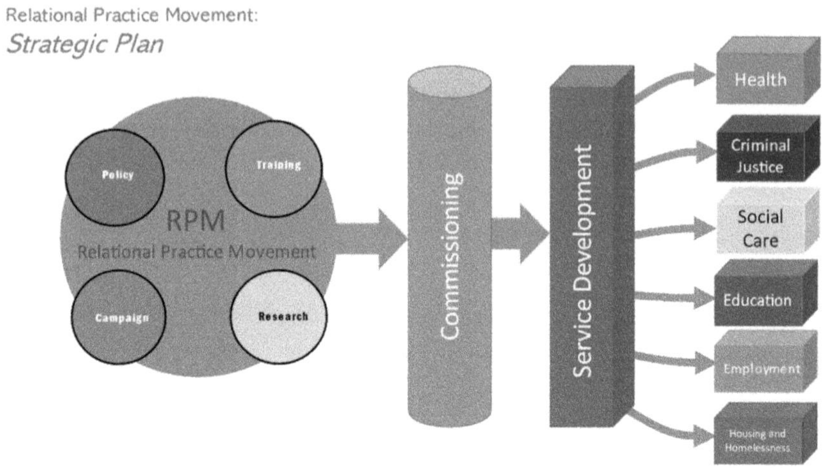

Fig. 14.4 Process for embedding relational practice across the public sector

A Manifesto

There is now a need for an active campaign to bring about change. The movement that has happened to date has raised professional awareness and found a high level of support amongst those with lived experience of services. The next step needs to be widespread consultations and a co-production process—across all organisations, professions and sectors—and coordination of an effective campaign to bring about these changes. The draft of a 'rallying call' manifesto, mostly taken from the text of this chapter, is presented in Fig. 14.5.

MANIFESTO

FOR A
RELATIONAL PRACTICE MOVEMENT

FOR TOO LONG PUBLIC SERVICES HAVE PURSUED A NARROW, MANAGERIAL PERFORMANCE FRAMEWORK: WITH THE UNINTENTIONAL CONSEQUENCES OF REDUCING ACCESS TO WHAT PEOPLE MOST NEED, AND REDUCING STAFF PERFORMANCE.

WE NEED A NEW VISION TO ENSURE THAT FACILITATIVE AND NON-TOXIC ENVIRONMENT ARE AVAILABLE IN ALL INTERACTIONS WITH, AND WITHIN, STATE-FUNDED AGENCIES TO MAKE THEM MORE HELPFUL THAN HARMFUL.

RELATIONAL PRACTICE GIVES PRIORITY TO RELATIONSHIPS OVER PROCEDURE AND IS THE FOUNDATION UPON WHICH EFFECTIVE INTERVENTIONS ARE MADE.
IT FORMS THE CONDITIONS FOR A HEALTHY AND ENABLING ENVIRONMENT.

IT IS THE ANTIDOTE TO DEHUMANISATION, COMMODIFICATION AND THE LOSS OF HUMAN DIGNITY AND AGENCY.

Fig. 14.5 Statements from this chapter incorporated into a draft 'manifesto'

References

Auty, K. M., & Liebling, A. (2020). Exploring the relationship between prison social climate and reoffending. *Justice Quarterly, 37*(2), 358–381.

Bellis, M. A., Ashton, K., Hughes, K., Ford, K. J., Bishop, J., & Paranjothy, S. (2016). *Adverse childhood experiences and their impact on health-harming behaviours in the Welsh adult population*. Public Health Wales NHS Trust.

Benefield, N., Turner, K., Bolger, L., & Bainbridge, C. (2017). Psychologically informed planned environments: A new optimism for criminal justice provision? In *Transforming environments and rehabilitation* (pp. 179–197). Routledge.

Bion, W. R. (1985). Container and contained. *Group Relations Reader, 2*(8), 127–133.

Bowlby, J. (2008). *A secure base: Parent-child attachment and healthy human development*. Basic Books.

Bradley, K. J. C. B. (2009). The Bradley Report: Lord Bradley's review of people with mental health problems or learning disabilities in the criminal justice system. Department of Health London.

Castillo, H. (2003). *Personality disorder: Temperament or trauma? An account of an emancipatory research study carried out by service users diagnosed with personality disorder* (Vol. 23). Jessica Kingsley Publishers.

Coid, J., Yang, M., Bebbington, P., Moran, P., Brugha, T., Jenkins, R., Farrell, M., Singleton, N., & Ullrich, S. (2009). Borderline personality disorder: Health service use and social functioning among a national household population. *Psychological Medicine, 39*(10), 1721–1731.

Council, K. C. (2006). *Report of the independent inquiry into the care and treatment of Michael Stone*.

Crawford, M., Rutter, D., Price, K., Weaver, T., Josson, M., Tyrer, P., Gibson, S., Gillespie, S., Faulkner, A., & Ryrie, I. (2007). *Learning the lessons: A multi-method evaluation of dedicated community-based services for people with personality disorder*. National Co-Ordinating Centre for NHS Service Delivery & Organisation, Journal Article. http://www.netscc.ac.uk/hsdr/files/project/SDO_FR_08-1404-083_V01.pdf

Daston, L. (2022). *Rules: A short history of what we live by* (Vol. 23). Princeton University Press.

Department of Health. (2009). Recognising complexity: Commissioning guidance for personality disorder services. *Journal Article*.

Engel, G. L. (1980). The clinical application of the biopsychosocial model. *American Journal of Psychiatry, 137*(5), Article 5.

Foulkes, S. H. (1983). *Introduction to group analytic psychotherapy: Studies in the social integration of individuals and groups*. Karnac Books.

Haigh, R. (2000). Support systems. 2. Staff sensitivity groups. *Advances in Psychiatric Treatment, 6*(4), 312–319.

Haigh, R. (2004). The quintessence of an effective team: Some developmental dynamics for staff groups. In *From toxic institutions to therapeutic environments* (pp. 119–130).

Haigh, R. (2007). The 16 personality disorder pilot projects. *Mental Health Review Journal, 12*(4), 29–39.

Haigh, R. (2013). The quintessence of a therapeutic environment. *Therapeutic Communities: The International Journal of Therapeutic Communities, 34*(1), 6–15.

Haigh, R., & Benefield, N. (2019). Towards a unified model of human development. *MH Review Journal, 24*(2), 124–132.

Haigh, R., & Benefield, N. (2020). Personality disorder: Breakdown in the relational field. In *Working effectively with personality disorder: A paradigm shift* (pp. 35–52). Wiley.

Haigh, R., Harrison, T., Johnson, R., Paget, S., & Williams, S. (2012). Psychologically informed environments and the "Enabling Environments" initiative. *Housing, Care and Support, 15*(1), 34–42.

Horn, N., Johnstone, L., & Brooke, S. (2007). Some service user perspectives on the diagnosis of borderline personality disorder. *Journal of Mental Health, 16*(2), 255–269.

Lewis, G., & Appleby, L. (1988). Personality disorder: The patients psychiatrists dislike. *The British Journal of Psychiatry: The Journal of Mental Science, 153*(Journal Article), 44–49.

Maden, T. (2006). DSPD: Origins and progress to date. *The British Journal of Forensic Practice, 8*(4), 24–28.

National Institute for Mental Health in England. (2003). Personality disorder: No longer a diagnosis of exclusion. *Policy Implementation Guidance for the Development of Services for People with Personality Disorder*. Department of Health.

NICE. (2009a). *Antisocial personality disorder (CG77).* National Institute for Health and Clinical Excellence: Guidance.

NICE. (2009b). *Borderline personality disorder (CG78).* National Institute for Health and Clinical Excellence: Guidance. http://europepmc.org/books/NBK55403

NIMHE. (2003). *Breaking the cycle of rejection: The personality disorders capabilities framework*. DH.

Pearce, S., & Pickard, H. (2013). How therapeutic communities work: Specific factors related to positive outcome. *The International Journal of Social Psychiatry, 59*(7), 636–645. https://doi.org/10.1177/0020764012450992

Robinson, L., & Cox, V. (Eds.). (2006). *Voices beyond the border: Living with borderline personality disorder*. Chipmunka Publishing.

Royal College of Psychiatrists. (2016). *What is the Enabling Environments award?* https://tinyurl.com/EEatRCPsych

Shuker, R., & Newton, M. (2008). Treatment outcome following intervention in a prison-based therapeutic community: A study of the relationship between reduction in criminogenic risk and improved psychological well-being. *The British Journal of Forensic Practice, 10*(3), 33–44.

Sibbald, S. (2020). Life and labels: Some personal thoughts about personality disorder. In S. P. Joramsden & J. Blazdell (Eds.), *working effectively with personality disorder* (pp. 23–33). Pavilion.

Soeteman, D. I., Roijen, L. H., Verheul, R., & Busschbach, J. J. (2008). The economic burden of personality disorders in mental health care. *Journal of Clinical Psychiatry, 69*(2), 259.

Thomas, P., Bracken, P., Cutler, P., Hayward, R., May, R., & Yasmeen, S. (2005). Challenging the globalisation of biomedical psychiatry. *Journal of Public Mental Health, 4*(3), 23–32.

Trevillion, K., Stuart, R., Ocloo, J., Broeckelmann, E., Jeffreys, S., Jeynes, T., Allen, D., Russell, J., Billings, J., & Crawford, M. J. (2021). Service user perspectives of community mental health services for people with complex emotional needs: A co-produced qualitative interview study. *MedRxiv*.

Wilson, L., & Haigh, R. (2011). *Innovation in action*.

Winifred Bolton, Lovell, K., Morgan, L., & Wood, H. (2014). *Meeting the challenge, making a difference*. Department of Health.

Winnicott, D. W. (1965). *The maturational process and the facilitating environment*. Hogarth Press.

15

Concluding Thoughts: Relational Hopes, Relational Realities

Michael Larkin and Zoë Boden-Stuart

We hope that this book has provided some important and useful insights into the benefits of approaching mental health from a relational perspective. Our aim was to foreground lived experiences from various perspectives, while highlighting the roles that relationality can play in mental health experience, and pointing towards ways that services and society can support this in future. We hope that such a focus will contribute to the development of an ethical, values-led practice, centred around care, compassion and shared humanity. At times, mental health care can seem like it is a long way from such a focus, but we think that there are chapters in this book which provide glimpses of what that can look like, both inside and outside formal services, and we hope that it can be achieved.

One of the main challenges involved in the development and spread of relationally-focused work is that structurally, socially and organisationally,

M. Larkin (✉)
Aston University, Birmingham, UK
e-mail: m.larkin@aston.ac.uk

Z. Boden-Stuart
The Open University, Milton Keynes, UK

Z. Boden-Stuart, M. Larkin (eds.), *Relationships and Mental Health*,
https://doi.org/10.1007/978-3-031-50047-3_15

individualism is 'baked in.' In the introductory chapters to this book (Part I), we described how problems are typically situated as properties of individuals, and that services are typically designed to respond to those difficulties at the individual level. This is largely a reflection of how capitalist society is organised, but there are exceptions. In the UK and Australia, for example, post-partum mental health difficulties, such as depression and psychosis, are supported by Mother and Baby Units. Family therapy is often provided to children and young people experiencing a range of different mental health difficulties. Both these examples illustrate how there are precedents for focusing our care and attention on the relational system, rather than on the discrete individual. Relational interventions like these, along with attachment-based services and whole-family approaches are more common in children and young people's mental health care in the UK, but the transition to adult mental health care at 18 seems to mean an abrupt end to relational thinking in most areas of practice.

In Part II of the book our contributors argue that traumatic relational events require relational contexts for healing. The chapters in this part of the book focus on times of crisis and complexity, whether that's suicidal or psychosis-related crises, surviving sexual abuse, or the traumas implicated in being a refugee or asylum-seeker. Each chapter provides a different relational approach to support the healing and recovery of the person in distress: through reciprocity and care within a family and community system; through encountering a service based on relational values and determined to interrupt harmful relational patterns; and through the provision of a reparative psychotherapeutic relationship.

Part III of the book explored how people experience relationships at times of distress. Intimate and supportive relationships considered in this part of the book include those with parents, siblings, peers with shared experiences of distress, and community volunteers in a non-mental health setting. Each group, in their own way, is looking to help the person in distress, but these relationships are complex and nuanced. Peer relationships, founded on equality and mutuality, have been highly influential in mental health care. However, bringing peer support into mainstream mental health services has not been without its critics, and the nature of peer-to-peer support changes fundamentally when a third party, like a mental health institution, becomes involved. The relational values that underpin peer support in community and clinical settings need careful consideration to ensure it is a positive experience for all involved.

Family relationships in the context of mental health are perhaps especially complex, due in part to the entanglement between childhood adversity and poor mental health. Unlike professional or professionalised caring relationships, familial relationships are more vulnerable to the strain that explicit signs of distress bring into the system. Challenging emotions like guilt, shame and envy, anxiety and fear, can mean that psychological crisis and recovery are often painful for all involved. However, this is not to say that this emotional landscape only exists in the context of families. Where there is extreme distress, trauma or desperation, whether that's in a community or clinical setting, there will be complex intersubjective experiences. Handling these situations reflectively, with compassion, and affording dignity to all involved is what is at stake.

The chapters in Part IV of this book give a good overview of what happens when services struggle to handle a relational topic with humanity and compassion. Intimacies, particularly sex and romance, are particularly fraught issues for mental health services. Whilst sex is becoming less taboo in society more generally, there are still plenty of people and places where discussing sexual activities, desires and feelings are not welcomed. Mental health services seem to often be among these places, and there are institutional silences when it comes to caring about the intimacy needs of people recovering from mental health crises. Residential psychiatric facilities, such as secure forensic wards, have a particularly difficult time addressing the messy realities of their patients' sexualities. Equating sex and relationships more broadly with risk, and ignoring the potentially supportive and protective factors associated with close relationships, is commonplace across a range of services, but what is clear from the chapters in this book is that there are ways forward to improve how clinicians support people to safely navigate this fundamental aspect of personhood.

In this final section of the book, we look forward. Our contributors have shown us some of the many dimensions that can be and should be considered when we begin to think relationally about mental health. To fully embrace such a shift in focus requires something more substantive than simply expanding our capacity to deliver family therapy. A reframing of the way that systems orient towards mental distress is required—we may need a manifesto for change, such as the one provided by Haigh and Benefield in this section. Friesen (2022) has pointed out that it is instructive to compare social responses to psychotic crises and psychedelic emergencies. During a distressing psychotic episode, people are likely to find themselves isolated from others, probably detained, and perhaps restrained. During a psychedelic emergency, people are likely to find that someone takes care to stay with them during the period of distress and disorientation, and that they are supported with reassurance and compassion. As Friesen (2023) has pointed out, there are already approaches to mental health support which embrace these values (the Soteria movement, for example), but these tend to operate as marginal and notable exceptions in most OECD countries. It can be dispiriting to reflect upon the scale of change which is required—especially given that many of our post-pandemic care systems and resources are seriously depleted—but it is also possible to be hopeful.

However, we must also acknowledge the partial nature of our enterprise. In this book, for example, we have relatively little from an attachment perspective, and yet this is one of the most important theoretical frames in psychology (but see Berry et al., 2020, for extensive discussion of attachment and relationships). We have also said relatively little about the typical mental health benefits of friendships or of romantic relationships, and yet these are perhaps the most widely experienced types of positive relationship. The latter remains an underdeveloped area of research, perhaps because sociologists drawn towards the topic of mental health have tended to focus on the structural issues underpinning the inequalities involved, whilst psychologists have tended to focus on individual differences and on developing interventions. While the focus of chapters in this volume has generally foregrounded mental health as a distinctive context, we note that in *relational* terms the chapters have tended to assume relatively normative understandings of what relationships look like, and of how people and communities interact with mental health services. However, there are a wide range of intersectional complexities at play in people's relational lives, and in their relationships to services, and we have barely scratched the surface of those issues in this volume. And so there is more work to do, and many gaps in our knowledge which still need filling.

A related area for reflection is of course the degree of representativeness of the contributors to our book. We have contributions from both hemispheres (but only from OECD countries), so although the cultural perspectives on relationships and mental health here have some range, that range is limited. As noted above, there are also further theoretical and conceptual perspectives which do have important contributions to make to the literature. We have tried to engage with a wide range of disciplinary perspectives. In the 'Concepts' chapter we draw explicitly on various philosophical, psychiatric and social psychological perspectives. In later chapters, ideas from lived experience, counselling, psychotherapy, social work, forensic psychology and clinical psychology are also foregrounded. There is also the matter of chapters authored by experts-by-experience. We have one chapter explicitly written from that perspective, but there are others where this perspective is present, but managed differently. Identities are complex, and not everyone manages their authorial identity in the same way: some people with lived experience become formal researchers in academic institutions, and may prefer to foreground the latter identity, for example. Nevertheless, across all of these dimensions, we have been reflecting on what we might have done differently in order to enable a more diverse range of contributions to be included in the book.

There are not only gaps between different paradigms, disciplines, and stakeholders—there are tensions too. For example, when relationships are foregrounded, professionals working in statutory services often express concerns about risk, as we've described above in the case of intimacy. However, from the perspective of service-providers, one benefit of individualist models is that they rarely have to consider the involvement of third parties who are not constrained by professional standards. When they do have to engage with significant others, it is typically when an orientation towards risk is activated. It is impossible to take sensitivity to risk out of the equation altogether when professionals are responsible for others' safety and wellbeing, however, it may well be that additional, relationally-focused components need to be *added* to such calculations.

There are many problems we face that are not amenable to 'human-scale' responses, but the development of relationally-oriented adult mental health care is not one of those problems. In our research and in our practice, we can make progress by being curious about the relational context of people's distress, and of their capacity to cope with it. When we train, supervise, innovate, coproduce, or evaluate, we can incorporate a relational perspective into our plans. We can grow the community of people who are mindful of a relational focus through praxis. Coproduction is an interesting example in this context. The proliferation and acceptance of coproduction and codesign in research and service development can be seen as a good example of how an innovation can spread and develop through practice. Due to its prevalence, coproduction is now also a potential mechanism for highlighting many of the important positive aspects of relational working. Collective action leads to change.

Some of the things that might improve the relational response to mental health difficulties may include policies that encourage investment in relational benefits over the long term. This would involve investing in the kinds of preventative public health initiatives (much as the Surestart[1] programme once did) that support relational capacities during the early years of development. However, it would also mean investing in local infrastructure and other forms of community-based social capital that can reduce loneliness and social distance in the shorter term. During the first year of the Covid-19 pandemic, many communities organised themselves in such ways (developing mutual aid strategies to support vulnerable or isolated community members). While much of the momentum has now been lost, there are still structures and relationships which remain, and which could be nurtured through further support and investment.

At the level of professional skills, it would be helpful to provide more consistent basic training across all professions on communication and relationship-building (e.g. see Bergen et al., 2022 during clinical encounters). To take this further, services could then develop and provide training on how to incorporate relational strengths and needs into mental health assessments, and—crucially—on working *with* service-users to

---

[1] SureStart is a British initiative aimed at parents and young children. Funding cuts led to SureStart centres being drastically reduced in number over the last ten years.

decide how and when to incorporate those strengths into treatment and support plans.

At a service level, there is a need at a national level, to codevelop and sustain new services to provide information and support to friends, family and other informal caregivers, in order that a relational shift is not simply a means to 'offload' care onto others. Co-developed resources are needed that help services structure their policies for thinking about risk in the context of the growing relational aspects of care. More specifically, it remains crucial that crisis and acute services are delivered in ways which are more equitable, accessible, and transparent, less coercive, and thus more likely to be trusted. Finally, we might suggest that providing pathways to care which are better supported by information from others who have accessed that care (i.e. relational insights), would allow people to find their way more easily to the right interventions and services for them.

References

Bergen, C., Bortolotti, L., Tallent, K., Broome, M., Larkin, M., Temple, R., Fadashe, C., Lee, C., Lim, M. C., & McCabe, R. (2022). Communication in youth mental health clinical encounters: Introducing the agential stance. *Theory & Psychology, 32*, 667. https://doi.org/10.1177/09593543221095079

Berry, K., Bucci, S., & Danquah, A. N. (Eds.). (2020). *Attachment theory and psychosis: Current perspectives and future directions*. Routledge.

Friesen, P. (2022). Psychosis and psychedelics: Historical entanglements and contemporary contrasts. *Transcultural Psychiatry, 59*(5), 592–609. https://doi.org/10.1177/13634615221129116

Friesen, P. (2023). *Psychosis and psychedelics: Historical entanglements and contemporary contrasts*. Too mad to be true II - The promises and perils of the first-person perspective. Sunday May 28, 2023. Museum Dr. Guislain, Gent.

Index[1]

[1] Note: Page numbers followed by 'n' refer to notes.

Z. Boden-Stuart, M. Larkin (eds.), *Relationships and Mental Health*,
https://doi.org/10.1007/978-3-031-50047-3

F

I

L

P

R

S

GPSR Compliance

The European Union's (EU) General Product Safety Regulation (GPSR) is a set of rules that requires consumer products to be safe and our obligations to ensure this.

If you have any concerns about our products, you can contact us on

ProductSafety@springernature.com

In case Publisher is established outside the EU, the EU authorized representative is:

Springer Nature Customer Service Center GmbH
Europaplatz 3
69115 Heidelberg, Germany

www.ingramcontent.com/pod-product-compliance
Ingram Content Group UK Ltd.
Pitfield, Milton Keynes, MK11 3LW, UK
UKHW020834290926
15470UKWH00004B/1343
* 9 7 8 3 0 3 1 5 0 0 4 6 6 *